KIDNEY DISEASES

DIET

THE DOCTOR'S DIAGNOSIS!

STOPPING RENAL DISTURBS THANKS TO LOW

SODIUM & POTASSIUM HEALTHY RECIPES

Written by **SIMON LEE**

Congratulation on purchase this book and thank You for doing so.

Please enjoy

© Copyright 2019 by **SIMON LEE**

reader. Under no circumstances will any legal responsibility or blame be held against the publisher for any reparation, damages, or monetary loss due to the information herein, either directly or indirectly.

Respective authors own all copyrights not held by the publisher.

The information herein is offered for informational purposes solely and is universal as so. The presentation of the information is without a contract or any guarantee assurance.

The trademarks that are used are without any consent, and the publication of the trademark is without permission or backing by the trademark owner. All trademarks and brands within this book are for clarifying purposes only and are owned by the owners themselves, not affiliated with this document.

PRINTED IN USA

CONTENTS

INTRODUCTION

A number of diseases can affect the kidneys.

Medical or ecological factors might result in kidney disease, and they can trigger functional and structural issues from birth in some people.

Reabsorption of nutrients

The kidneys reabsorb nutrients from the blood and transfer them to where they would best support health.

They also reabsorb other products to help maintain homeostasis.

Reabsorbed items consist of:

- Water.
- Phosphate.
- Bicarbonate.
- Glucose.
- Amino Acids.
- Salt.

–   Chloride, Salt, Potassium, And Magnesium Ions.

Secretion of active substances.

The kidneys launch a variety of important substances, including:

Erythropoietin: This controls erythropoiesis or the production of red cells. The liver likewise produces erythropoietin, but the kidneys are its main producers in grownups.

Renin: These assist in managing the expansion of arteries and the volume of blood plasma, lymph, and interstitial fluid. Lymph is a fluid that contains leukocyte, which supports immune activity, and interstitial fluid is the primary part of extracellular fluid.

Calcitriol: This is the hormonally active metabolite of vitamin D. It increases both the quantity of calcium that the intestinal tracts can absorb and the reabsorption of phosphate in the kidney.

Managing blood pressure.

The kidneys control high blood pressure when required. However, they are accountable for slower changes.

They adjust long-term pressure in the arteries by triggering changes in the fluid outside of cells. The medical term for this fluid is extracellular fluid.

These fluid modifications take place after the release of a vasoconstrictor called angiotensin II. Vasoconstrictors are hormonal agents that trigger blood vessels to narrow.

They deal with other functions to increase the kidneys' absorption of sodium chloride or salt. This effectively increases the size of the extracellular fluid compartment and raises blood pressure.

Anything that alters high blood pressure can harm the kidneys with time, consisting of extreme alcohol obesity, smoking, and usage.

Waste excretion

The kidneys remove a number of waste items and eliminate them in the urine. 2 major substances that the kidneys eliminate are:

- urea, which arises from the breakdown of proteins
- uric acid from the breakdown of nucleic acids

Diabetic nephropathy.

In people with diabetic nephropathy, damage happens to the capillaries of the kidney as an outcome of long-lasting diabetes.

Symptoms do not end up being clear until years after the damage starts to establish.

They consist of:

- Inflamed Legs.
- Nausea.
- Tiredness.

- Headaches.
- Scratchy Skin.

The kidneys are one of the more vital tissues examined. Because of its function in the purification, metabolic process, and excretion of substances, it is often the site of test-article-induced lesions. In addition, a vast array of spontaneous renal lesions might be observed. Chronic progressive nephropathy (CPN), an age-related and spontaneous disease of rodents, may be worsened by chemical administration and is a confounding aspect in the analysis of renal toxicology and carcinogenic findings.

The kidneys are a pair of bean-shaped organs present in all vertebrates. They eliminate waste items from the body, keep well-balanced electrolyte levels, and regulate blood pressure.

The kidneys are some of the most important organs. The Ancient Egyptians left only the brain and kidneys in position before embalming a body, inferring that they held a higher worth.

Keeping pH

In people, the acceptable pH level is between 7.38 and 7.42. Listed below this limit, the body goes into a state of acidemia, and above it, alkalemia.

Outside this range, enzymes and proteins break down and can no longer function. In severe cases, this can be fatal.

The kidneys and lungs assist in keeping a steady pH within the body. The lungs achieve this by moderating the concentration of CO_2.

The kidneys manage the pH through 2 procedures:

Reabsorbing and regenerating bicarbonate from urine: Bicarbonate helps reduce the effects of acids. If the pH is tolerable or launch it if acid levels rise, the kidneys can either maintain it.

Excreting hydrogen ions and fixed acids: Fixed or nonvolatile acids are any acids that do not occur as an outcome of CO_2. They arise from the insufficient metabolic process of proteins, carbs, and fats. They consist of lactic acid, sulfuric acid, and phosphoric acid.

Kidney stones

Stones can form a solid accumulation of minerals in the kidney.

If they obstruct the ureter, they can trigger extreme discomfort and might impact kidney function.

Structure

The kidneys are at the back of the stomach cavity, with one resting on each side of the spine.

The ideal kidney is usually somewhat smaller sized and lower than the left, to make area for the liver.

Each kidney weighs 125-- 170 grams (g) in males and 115-- 155 g in females.

A tough, fibrous kidney capsule surrounds each kidney. Beyond that, 2 layers of fat work as protection. The adrenal glands lay on top of the kidneys.

Inside the kidneys are a number of pyramid-shaped lobes. These are the urine-producing structures of the kidneys.

Blood goes into the kidneys through the kidney arteries and leaves through the renal veins. The kidneys are reasonably little organs however, receive 20-- 25 percent of the heart's output.

Each kidney excretes urine through a tube called the ureter that results in the bladder.

Function

The primary function of the kidneys is preserving homeostasis. This indicates they manage fluid levels, electrolyte balance, and other factors that keep the internal environment of the body comfortable and constant.

They serve a broad range of functions.

Causes

Neck and back pain is a symptom of kidney damage.

Back discomfort is a symptom of kidney damage.

Some of the most typical reasons for kidney damage consist of:

- Lithium: Doctors prescribe lithium to deal with schizophrenia and bipolar disease. Lithium might trigger nephropathy with long-lasting use. Regardless of the risk, a person can avoid the negative effects of lithium with close medical guidance.

- Chemotherapy representatives: The most common type of kidney problem in people with cancer is severe kidney injury. This might be due to the extreme throwing up and diarrhea that are typical negative effects of chemotherapy.

- IgA nephropathy: Also known as Berger's disease, this takes place when immunoglobin A (IgA) antibodies build up in the kidney. It can result in kidney failure.

- Analgesics: Using discomfort medication over an extended period of time might result in chronic analgesic nephritis. Examples include aspirin, acetaminophen, and non-steroidal anti-inflammatory drugs (NSAIDs).

- Alcohol: Alcohol changes the kidneys' ability to filter the blood. It likewise dehydrates the body, making it harder for kidneys to redress internal balances, and increases blood pressure, which can likewise impede the kidneys.

Kidney tumor

These can be benign or deadly. Benign cancers do not spread out or attack tissue; however malignant cancers can be aggressive.

The most typical malignant kidney cancer is renal cell carcinoma.

Renal failure

In individuals with renal failure, the kidneys end up being not able to filter out waste items from the blood effectively.

If an injury causes kidney failure, such as the overuse of medication, the condition is typically reversible with treatment.

If the cause is an disease, however, kidney failure typically does not have a full treatment.

Kidney hydronephrosis

This suggests "water on the kidney."

It generally takes place when an obstruction prevents urine from leaving the kidney, causing extreme pain.

In time, the kidney may atrophy, or diminish.

Interstitial nephritis

A reaction to bacteria or medications can inflame the areas within the kidney.

Treatment normally involves eliminating the reason for swelling or altering a course of medication.

Duplicated ureter

Two ureters might form in between a kidney and the bladder, instead of one. There are a couple of issues, but it can increase the danger of urinary system infections and, in women, incontinence.

Duplicated ureter affects around 1 percent of individuals.

Kidney infections

These tend to arise from germs in the bladder that transfer to the kidneys.

Signs include lower pain in the back, unpleasant urination, and in some cases, fever. Changes in the urine may consist of the existence of blood, cloudiness, and a different odor.

Kidney infections are more typical in ladies than in males, as well as in ladies who are pregnant. The infection typically responds well to antibiotics.

Nephrotic syndrome

Damage to the kidney function triggers protein levels in the urine to increase. This results in a protein scarcity throughout the body, which draws water into the tissues.

Signs include:

- Puffy Eyes

- Increased Cholesterol Levels

- Fluid In The Lungs

- Anemia.

Changes in urination and lower pain in the back, especially on one side, might be indications of kidney issues.

Dialysis.

In the case of serious kidney damage, dialysis might be a choice. It is only used for end-stage kidney failure, where 85 to 90 percent of kidney function is lost.

Kidney dialysis intends to complete a few of the functions of a healthy kidney.

These include:

- Preserving the proper levels of chemicals in the blood, consisting of potassium, bicarbonate, and salt.

- Removal of waste, excess salt, and water.

- Keeping blood pressure.

The two most typical kinds of kidney dialysis are:

Hemodialysis: An artificial kidney, or hemodialyzer, removes waste, extra fluids, and chemicals. The treating physician makes an entry point in the body by connecting an artery and a vein under the skin to produce a bigger capillary.

Blood takes a trip into the hemodialyzer, gets treatment, and after that, goes back to the body. This is typically done 3 to 4 times a week. More routine dialysis has a more beneficial result.

Peritoneal dialysis: The physician inserts a sterilized service consisting of glucose into the stomach cavity around the intestinal tract. This is the peritoneum, and a protective membrane surrounds it.

The peritoneal membrane filters waste products as excess fluids go into the stomach cavity.

In continuous peritoneal dialysis, the fluid drains pipes through a catheter — the private discards these fluids 4 to 5 times a day. In automated peritoneal dialysis, the procedure occurs over time.

THE HISTORY OF KIDNEY DISEASE

In the twentieth century, private investigators such as Homer Smith revealed the underlying physiology of the kidney. Smith's searchings for brought about essential medical therapies for multiple kidney conditions. As technology boosted, therapy in the field of nephrology was additionally progressed with the initial effective usage of hemodialysis in 1945 by Willem Kolff. Quickly after that, in 1954, the initial effective kidney hair transplant was carried out in twins in Boston by Joseph E. Murray. With more work in immunology, Murray, as well as his team, were later able to transplant kidneys right into unassociated recipients with the usage of immunosuppressive treatment. Among the first effective situation, series-defining making use of immunosuppression (azathioprine or 6-mercaptopurine and glucocorticoids) was reported in the New England Journal of Medicine in 1963 by Murray and also coworkers.

The all-natural history of persistent kidney disease (CKD), in basic, continues to be conjectural. In 1666 individuals in the Modification of Diet in Renal Disease study, a much greater ESRD price of 60% after 88 months was reported (four times the fatality price); amongst clients older than 65 years, the fatality rate approximated the ESRD price. A 72-month prospective record of an aging associate of 100 CKD clients, great danger because they all experienced intense kidney injury at research access, is presented.

Chronic kidney disease (CKD) is a condition defined by a steady loss of kidney function with time.

What Is Persistent Kidney Disease (CKD)?

Persistent kidney disease consists of problems that damage your kidneys and also lower their ability to keep you healthy and balanced by doing the work provided. If kidney condition worsens, wastes can develop to high levels in your blood as well as make you really feel unwell. You might create difficulties like high blood stress, anemia (reduced blood matter), weak bones, bad dietary health, and wellness as well as nerve damages. The kidney condition raises your risk of having heart as well as blood vessel condition. These troubles might happen slowly over a long period of time. Chronic kidney disease might be triggered by diabetes, hypertension and also other problems. Early discovery, as well as treatment, can typically maintain chronic kidney condition from getting worse. When kidney condition progresses, it might at some point cause kidney failure, which calls for dialysis or a kidney transplant to keep life.

Today, medical nephrology remains to advance with lots of kinds of renal replacement therapy-- both acute and chronic-- consisting of hemodialysis, peritoneal dialysis, hemofiltration as well as hemodiafiltration, using erythropoietin for anemia in persistent kidney disease, therapy of renal osteodystrophy, ongoing renovations in immunosuppression for transplant, and also specific treatments for many nephropathies.

The initial acknowledgment of kidney disease as independent from various other clinical problems is widely credited to Richard Bright's 1827 publication "Reports of Medical Cases," which outlined the features and also consequences of a kidney condition. For the following 100 years approximately, the term "Bright's disease" was used to refer to any kind of kidney disease. Bright's findings led to the prevalent method of testing urine for protein-- one of the initial analysis tests in medication.

The study of kidney disease was enhanced by William Howship Dickinson's summary of severe nephritis in 1875 and Frederick Akbar Mahomed's discovery of the link between kidney condition as well as hypertension in the 1870s. Mahomed's original sphygmograph, developed when he was a medical student, was improved in 1896 by Scipione Riva-Rocci, of Italy, with the usage of a cuff to surround the arm.

Other problems that affect the kidneys are:

    –   Obstructions triggered by issues like kidney stones, tumors, or a bigger prostate gland in guys.

    –   Malformations that take place as an infant establishes in its mom's womb. A constricting might happen that avoids regular discharge of pee as well as creates pee to move back up to the kidney. This creates infections as well as may damage the kidneys.

–   Glomerulonephritis, a team of diseases that cause swelling and damage to the kidney's filtering system systems. These conditions are the third most typical kind of kidney condition.

–   Lupus, as well as various other diseasees that influence the body's immune system.

–   Inherited diseases, such as polycystic kidney condition, which causes big cysts to create in the kidneys and damage the surrounding cells.

–   Repeated urinary system infections.

What Are The Symptoms Of CKD?

Most individuals might not have any kind of serious signs up until their kidney disease is advanced. Nevertheless, you may notice that you:

- Have a poor appetite.
- Have puffy feet and ankle joints.
- Feel more tired and also have less power.
- Have puffiness around your eyes, particularly in the early morning.
- Have dry, itchy skin.
- Have muscle mass cramping during the night.
- Have trouble resting.
- Have difficulty focusing.
- The requirement to pee much more commonly, particularly during the night.
- The Facts About Chronic Kidney Disease (CKD).

–   African Americans, Hispanics, Pacific Islanders, American Indians, as well as Seniors are at enhanced danger.

–   Glomerular purification price (GFR) is the most effective price quote for kidney features.

–   High danger teams consist of those with diabetes mellitus, family members as well as high blood pressure history of kidney failure.

–   37 million American grownups have CKD, and numerous others go to enhanced risk.

–   Persistent proteinuria (protein in the urine) means CKD is existing.

–   Hypertension triggers CKD, and CKD causes high blood pressure.

–   Heart disease is the major reason for death for all individuals with CKD.

–   Early discovery can assist avoid the progression of kidney disease to kidney failure.

–   Two simple examinations can detect CKD: high blood pressure, pee albumin, and product creatinine.

What Creates CKD?

The two main reasons for chronic kidney disease are diabetic issues as well as high blood pressure, which are responsible for up to two-thirds of the cases. If uncontrolled or poorly regulated, high blood pressure can be a leading cause of heart strikes, strokes, and persistent kidney disease.

Any person can get chronic kidney disease at any age. Nonetheless, some individuals are more probable than others to establish kidney condition. You might have a boosted risk for kidney disease if you:

- Are older.
- Have hypertension.
- Have a family history of kidney failure.
- Have diabetes mellitus.
- Come from a population team that has a high price of diabetic issues or hypertension, such as African Americans, Hispanic Americans, Asian, Pacific Islanders, as well as American Indians.

UNDERSTANDING KIDNEY FAILURE

A number of typical themes arose. Right here are the four point's kidneys patients most wish others would certainly understand.

Diabetic Nephropathy

Diabetes is an disease that keeps the body from using glucose (sugar) as it should. If glucose remains in your blood as opposed to damaging down, it can imitate a poisonous substance. Damage to the nephrons from unused glucose in the blood is called diabetic person nephropathy. You can delay or prevent diabetic nephropathy if you keep your blood glucose levels down.

Many kidney diseases attack the nephrons, creating them to lose their filtering system ability. Many kidney diseases attack both kidneys all at once.

The most typical root causes of kidney disease are diabetes mellitus and also high blood pressure. If your family has a background of any kind of type of kidney troubles, you may go to threat for kidney disease.

Glomerular Diseases

A number of different kinds of kidney disease are grouped together under this category, consisting of autoimmune conditions, infection-related diseases as well as sclerotic diseases. As the name indicates, glomerular disease attack the little capillary (glomeruli) within the kidney.

The most typical main glomerular diseases consist of membranous nephropathy, IgA nephropathy, as well as focal segmental glomerulosclerosis. Protein, blood, or both in the urine are usually the very first indicators of this disease. They can gradually damage kidney features. High blood pressure control is essential with any kidney condition.

Therapies for glomerular conditions might include immunosuppressive medicines or steroids to decrease inflammation as well as proteinuria, relying on a certain disease.

Inherited as well as Congenital Kidney Diseases

Some kidney conditions result from hereditary elements. Polycystic kidney disease (PKD), as an example, is a congenital disease in which numerous cysts expand in the kidneys. PKD cysts can gradually replace much of the mass of the kidneys, lowering kidney features and also resulting in kidney failure.

The indicators of kidney disease in kids vary. Some kidney diseases may be "silent" for months or even years.

Your kid's physician must locate it during a normal appointment if your kid has kidney disease. Be sure your youngster sees a doctor frequently. The first sign of a kidney issue might be hypertension, a low variety of red cells (anemia), or blood or protein in the kid's urine.

If the physician finds any one of these problems, additionally examinations might be required, including added blood and also urine tests or radiology researches. Sometimes, the physician might require to do a biopsy-- eliminating a small piece of the kidney to check out under a microscope.

Some hereditary kidney disease may not be discovered until adulthood. The most common kind of PKD was when called "grown-up PKD" due to the fact that the symptoms of hypertension and renal failure usually do not occur until people remain in their 20s or 30s. With advancements in analysis imaging modern technology, physicians have actually found cysts in kids as well as teenagers prior to any type of signs show up.

Various Other Causes of Kidney Disease

Poisonous substances, as well as trauma, such as a direct and powerful blow to your kidneys, can bring about kidney disease. Some over the counter medicines can be harmful to your kidneys if taken consistently over a long period of time. Products that incorporate aspirin, acetaminophen, and also other medications such as Advil have actually been discovered to be the most harmful to the kidneys.

Things You Should Understand About Living with Kidney Disease:

A basic inquiry--"What do you want others recognized regarding coping with kidney condition?"-- let loose a gush of comments on our Facebook page lately. Kidney disease itself is often invisible up until the late stages; as soon as it progresses to kidney failure, individuals need dialysis or a transplant to live. Individuals coping with kidney disease and kidney failing tell us they usually really feel that they do not recognize what they are experiencing, both physically and psychologically.

Check with your physician to make sure you are not putting your kidneys in danger if you take medicines on a regular basis.

Hypertension

Hypertension can harm the small capillary in your kidneys. The harmed vessels cannot filter wastes from your blood as they are intended to.

Your physician may recommend blood pressure medication. Blood stress medicines called angiotensin-converting enzyme (ACE) inhibitors and also angiotensin receptor blockers (ARBs) have actually been located to secure the kidneys a lot more than other medicines that reduced high blood pressure to similar levels.

The National Heart, Lung, and also Blood Institute (NHLBI), among the National Institutes of Health, recommends that people with diabetic issues or lowered kidney function should maintain their high blood pressure below 130/80 mm Hg.

1. It's laborious

There's a special type of weary that frequently accompanies kidney disease, and it's not constantly foreseeable. "I have my excellent days and also my poor," keep in mind Emily. "Some days, I desire to rest as well as most I'm prepared to go." For lots of, the fatigue is prevalent. "I'm not careless," states Linda. "My energy level resembles a person at the end of a complete day of job when I get up." Valerie composes, "I'm always tired! As well as I believe my household and also good friends obtain tired of hearing that." Some individuals compare it to the flu: "It's like really feeling flulike weary all the time as well as not thinking plainly because you're so exhausted," states Lori. Emily summarizes what individuals desire: "Most of all, all we want is understanding, persistence, and approval."

2. Looks can be deceiving

Kidney disease does not have outside physical signs, so close friends, coworkers, and also family members may have a difficult time comprehending simply how inadequately people typically really feel. "Just since I look OK does not imply I feel ALRIGHT," composes Natalie. Lots of people make maintaining up with their appearance a top priority: "I always attempt to put on a 'typical' as well as 'healthy and balanced' look when I leave the house," creates Jill.

3. The pain is genuine

The pain that usually comes with kidney disease and also dialysis treatments can make it tough to do lots of things healthy individuals consider granted. "The pain never stops," creates Heather Marie. "Even choosing my children up to hold them hurts as well as nobody might understand that sort of pain." Notes Delores: "Even the smallest simplest points are difficult to do, and also the discomfort and exhaustion, especially the day after dialysis. And also, dialysis is excruciating. You are not simply resting there for 3-4 hours enjoying yourself with 2 big needles stuck in your arm." Michelle uses this advice: "Be helpful and also recognize we deal with some type of discomfort daily, in some cases, extreme."

4. There is no remedy

When the kidneys have fallen short, the only treatments are dialysis or transplant. "Dialysis is not a cure," writes Kevin. "It is, for all intents and also objectives, a life-sustaining therapy. Which is all." JeJe states, "Not even a transplant will certainly make you healthy and balanced. Your life is simply maintained with medications and also extreme therapies."

Regardless of these obstacles, numerous clients inform us they function hard to preserve a positive overview and live their lives to the fullest. And they want others to stay clear of experiencing what they are: "A LOT of individuals with kidney condition do not even understand they have it," writes Roselie. "Get evaluated!"

CAUSES OF KIDNEY DISEASE OR KIDNEY FAILURE

Kidney condition is rather a danger to your general health due to the function your kidneys play in a large range of important bodily functions. Damages normally establish gradually over a long duration of time. Just one kidney may be influenced, yet typically, damage happens in both.

Signs and symptoms commonly don't show up until it has actually advanced to a dangerous phase. As a matter of fact, kidneys can maintain functioning when only 15 percent of normal feature stays, and there will certainly be a few signs that anything serious is incorrect.

Chronic kidney disease, also called chronic kidney failure, defines the steady loss of kidney function. Your kidneys filter wastes and also excess fluids from your blood, which are then secreted in your urine.

When persistent kidney condition gets to an innovative phase, dangerous levels of liquid, wastes, and electrolytes can develop in your body.

Therapy for chronic kidney disease focuses on slowing down the progression of kidney damage, usually by managing the underlying reason. Chronic kidney disease can proceed to end-stage kidney failure, which is fatal without a man-made filtering system (dialysis) or a kidney transplant.

Diabetic issues and also high blood pressure are the most usual sources of chronic kidney disease (CKD). Your healthcare carrier will certainly take a look at your health history and also might do tests to discover why you have kidney disease. The root cause of your kidney disease may influence the kind of treatment you obtain.

Persistent kidney disease occurs when an disease or condition harms kidney features, triggering kidney damage to intensify over a number of months or years.

High blood pressure

High blood stress can damage capillary in the kidneys, so they do not work too. If the capillary in your kidneys is damaged, your kidneys may not work as well to eliminate wastes and additional liquid from your body. Additional fluid in the blood vessels might then elevate high blood pressure also more, producing an unsafe cycle.

Other reasons for a kidney condition

- IgA glomerulonephritis
- a drug that is harmful to the kidneys
- An disease that impacts the entire body, such as diabetic issues or lupus Lupus nephritis is the medical name for kidney condition brought on by lupus.
- Other reasons for kidney disease include
- uncommon genetic problems, such as Alport syndrome
- A congenital disease that creates several cysts to expand in the kidneys, polycystic kidney disease (PKD).

–   an infection

–   heavy metal poisoning, such as lead poisoning

–   Henoch-Schönlein purpura

–   hemolytic uremic disorder in kids

–   conditions in which the body's immune system strikes its very own cells and also body organs, such as Goodpasture syndrome

–   renal artery constriction

In the very early phases of persistent kidney disease, you may have few indicators or signs. Chronic kidney disease may not emerge up until your kidney function is dramatically impaired.

Diabetic issues

Excessive sugar, likewise called sugar, in your blood damages your kidneys' filters. Gradually, your kidneys can end up being so harmed that they no more do a good task filtering wastes and additional liquid from your blood.

Usually, the first indication of kidney disease from diabetes mellitus is healthy protein in your pee. When the filters are damaged, a protein called albumin, which you require to remain healthy, loses consciousness of your blood as well as right into your urine. A healthy and balanced kidney does not let albumin pass from the blood into the urine.

Diabetic kidney disease is the medical term for kidney disease caused by diabetes.

The Most Common Causes of Kidney Disease

Complications.

Persistent kidney disease can impact virtually every component of your body. Potential complications might consist of:

Clearly, kidney condition can be an extremely hazardous issue for any individual that has diabetes.

Hypertension

High blood stress puts excess force on cells and also tissues as blood comes with. This decreases function and also effectiveness by the kidneys as a whole.

Family Members History

When it comes to having kidney issues, genes appear to matter. If a lot of people in your family members has actually had a kidney problem, you are most likely at greater danger of having it too.

Foods You Eat

What you consume can make a big distinction in kidney wellness. If your daily diet plan consists of a wealth of meat and also healthy protein, your opportunity of having kidney condition is above standard.

Salt

The quantity of salt (salt) in your diet likewise matters. While it's real that you require salt, eating excessively of it threatens your kidneys. And keep in mind, salt not just comes from the salt shaker at the household supper table, but likewise exists in large amounts in processed dinner mixes, potato chips, salted nut snacks, cold cuts, several sorts of cheese, tinned and also immediate or dried soups, canned veggies and also bacon.

Any individual who is seriously concerned concerning kidney health and wellness and avoiding kidney condition will wish to keep the foods detailed over to a minimum.

Conditions and problems that cause chronic kidney disease include:

- Glomerulonephritis (gloe-mer-u-low-nuh-FRY-tis), an inflammation of the kidney's filtering system devices (glomeruli).
- Interstitial nephritis (in-tur-STISH-ul nuh-FRY-is), swelling of the kidney's tubules and also bordering structures.
- Polycystic kidney disease.
- Type 1 or type 2 diabetic issues
- High blood stress
- Prolonged obstruction of the urinary system tract, from problems such as enlarged prostate, kidney rocks as well as some cancers.
- Vesicoureteral (ves-ih-koe-yoo-REE-tur-ul) reflux, a condition that creates pee to back up right into your kidneys.
- Recurrent kidney infection likewise called pyelonephritis (pie-uh-low-nuh-FRY-tis).

–   Decreased sex drive, impotence, or reduced fertility.

–   Fluid retention, which can lead to swelling in your legs as well as arms, high blood pressure, or fluid in your lungs (lung edema).

–   Pericarditis, swelling of the saclike membrane layer that covers your heart (pericardium).

–   Weak bones and also a raised risk of bone cracks.

–   Anemia.

–   A sudden increase in potassium levels in your blood (hyperkalemia), which might impair your heart's ability to function as well as may be deadly.

–   Decreased immune reaction, which makes you a lot more prone to infection.

–   Pregnancy difficulties that carry threats for the mother as well as the developing fetus.

–   Damage to your central nerve system, which can create trouble focusing, personality changes, or seizures.

–   Heart as well as blood vessel (cardiovascular) disease.

–   Irreversible damage to your kidneys (end-stage kidney condition), eventually need either dialysis or a kidney transplant for survival.

Risk factors

Aspects that might boost your threat of chronic kidney disease include:

–   Smoking.

–   Abnormal kidney framework.

–   Obesity.

–   Family background of kidney disease.

–   High blood pressure.

–   Being African-American, Native American, or Asian-American.

–   Diabetes.

–   Heart and also blood vessel (cardio) disease.

–   Older age.

Kidney disease is more likely to happen in the complying with scenarios.

Diabetic issues

In diabetes mellitus instances, the human body does not use glucose or sugar, the method it should. When this takes place, sugar begins to act like a toxin, triggering the kidneys to function more challenging. As they stress, the all-natural filters in the kidneys become a lot more porous. This permits contaminants and wastes to stay in the body, developing a cycle of damages that might lead to kidney failure. Any person who has kidney failing must either have dialysis or a kidney transplant.

SIGNS OF KIDNEY FAILURE

On top of that, various other kidney troubles that are not infections, such as nephrotic disorder, can also offer with symptoms such as:

- Edema or puffiness in the face, abdominal area, or legs.
- Weight gain as a result of fluid retention.
- Hypertension.
- Fatigue.
- Unexplained weight reduction.

Pink, red, or brownish urine is an indication of visible blood in the pee, recognized as gross hematuria, which is a sign and symptom of nephritic disorder (see listed below). This problem needs clinical therapy, as well as the affected individual, should look for clinical assistance.

Kidney failure takes place when the kidneys can no much longer do their key feature, which is to filter waste, water as well as salt from the body. When the kidneys do not filter appropriately, the chemical make-up of the blood can become unbalanced. Numerous medical issues can trigger kidney failure consisting of problems in which the kidneys do not obtain sufficient blood to filter (e.g., as a result of an infection, use pain killers as well as relevant drugs, heart problem, serious dehydration or severe allergy), when there are direct damages to the kidneys (e.g., due to embolism in the capillaries and also arteries surrounding the kidneys, inflammation of the filters in the kidneys, swelling of the kidneys from a medication or infection or lupus) or when the pee drainage tubes come to be obstructed making it make sure that wastes cannot exit the body with the pee (e.g., as a result of kidney stones, a bigger prostate or blood clots in the urinary tract).

Recognizing the symptoms of kidney disease can help people spot it early sufficient to obtain therapy. Signs and symptoms can include:

The healthy and balanced kidneys function to eliminate added water as well as wastes, assistance regulate blood stress, maintain body chemicals in equilibrium, maintain bones strong, inform your body to make red cells and also assist children to grow generally. Persistent kidney disease (CKD) takes place when kidneys are no more able to clean contaminants as well as waste items from the blood as well as execute their features to complete capability. This can happen all of a sudden or with time.

General Indications Of Kidney Troubles

Although there are lots of sorts of kidney problems, many kidney infections, such as acute pyelonephritis, share typical symptoms. These include:

- Pink, brownish or red pee
- Nausea.
- Chills.
- Pus in the pee
- Pain or burning while urinating
- Foamy, frothy or sparkling pee
- Urinating regularly and/or urgently
- Bad-smelling or cloudy pee
- Fever.
- Back discomfort, flank pain, and/or groin discomfort.

The kidneys create part of the urinary system, among the body's major filtering systems. The majority of people have two kidneys, situated in the upper abdominal location in the direction of the muscular tissues of the back and also the side of the ribs. The kidneys create part of the urinary system together with ureters, the bladder as well as urethra. Kidney troubles impact the kidneys; however, because the system collaborates, the impacts of a kidney issue are often felt throughout the system.

Kidney troubles in grownups and teens are normally uneasy, yet can commonly be treated relatively quickly by doctors. Because of the result, they can have on both the pregnant female and the infant, kidney troubles in expectant women are of particular concern. Diagnosing kidney problems in toddlers as well as children can be difficult due to the fact that their kidneys and also bodies are relatively smaller sized and also usually cannot clarify to their caretakers exactly how they are feeling or where they are harming.

Foamy pee is an indicator of proteinuria, which commonly also comes with swelling in the hands, feet, abdomen, and/or face. Proteinuria is a sign and symptom of nephrotic syndrome (see below).

The kidneys themselves cleanse the blood by filtering it in the nephrons, which are composed of a renal corpuscle and also a kidney tubule. The corpuscle is composed of a glomerulus confined by the Bowman's capsule. To filter the blood, it is gone through the glomeruli at higher stress than the body's usual blood pressure. Filtered waste items collect inside the Bowman's capsule, while filtered, clean blood is passed revoke the glomeruli into the blood circulation system. The tubule collects the waste items from the Bowman's capsule while additionally functioning on further trading specific substances as well as additionally reabsorbing water and specific minerals, so they don't go to waste. The resulting liquid is after that passed into the ureters as urine. Urine accumulates in the bladder, which stores it up until it is released by the urethra.

Greater than 37 million American grownups are dealing with a kidney condition, and also many don't know it. There are a number of physical indications of kidney disease, however often, individuals associate them with various other conditions. Those with kidney disease tend not to experience signs up until the extremely late phases, when the kidneys are failing or when there are huge amounts of protein in the urine. This is just one of the factors why just 10% of people with persistent kidney condition understand that they have it.

Signs Of Common Kidney Problems

In children, this kidney problem is usually brought on by a kidney problem referred to as minimal modification disease. Even more young boys than women are influenced, and many youngsters will experience the condition between the ages of 18 months and four years.

A diagnosis of chronic kidney condition is commonly made only in the later phases of the problem. In the beginning, the condition may not trigger disruptions that can be clinically measured. Signs and symptoms just show up later, and as soon as they do, the influenced person will certainly be examined by a medical professional to confirm that CKD exists.

Indicators Of Chronic Kidney Disease.

Persistent kidney disease (CKD) is normally without signs and also pain-free in its very early phases, other than in scenarios where an underlying condition causes discomfort. Persistent kidney condition takes a long period of time to create. If the affected individual's signs and symptoms develop over a variety of hrs or a few days, it is a lot more most likely that the kidney issue they are experiencing is severe kidney injury (see below).

In adults, nephrotic syndrome is frequently triggered by 2 kidney problems that are connected with, e.g., diabetes mellitus, autoimmune disorders such as systemic lupus erythematosus, or infections such as Hepatitis B or C, or HIV infection. Severe preeclampsia is a cause of nephrotic disorder in expectant ladies.

Signs and symptoms of nephrotic syndrome consist of:

–   Hypoalbuminemia, low levels of the protein albumin in the blood.

–   Edema or puffiness anywhere in the body, yet especially around the eyes.

–   Malaise and exhaustion.

–   High cholesterol.

–   High blood stress.

–   Loss of appetite.

–   Frothy urine.

–   Albuminuria, high degrees of albumin in the pee.

In females and also guys older than 65, the prior signs might be absent, and also added signs might consist of:

–   Jumbled speech.

–   Confusion.

–   Hallucinations.

If an older individual reveals signs and symptoms of kidney trouble, they must see a physician to have their kidney feature analyzed. For more information on the indications of age-related chronic kidney disease, see the area below.

Excellent to understand: In babies and kids, the only sign of intense pyelonephritis may be a high fever.

Proteinuria and edema are both the most distinct symptoms of the nephrotic disorder. Edema, specifically around the eyes, is just one of the first visible signs of nephrotic disorder.

Nephritic syndrome triggers the kidneys to be less effective at filtering waste compounds from the blood. In individuals with the nephritic disorder, protein and blood might be located in the urine. Nevertheless, most situations of the nephritic disorder are persistent and also have couple of signs and symptoms. The severe nephritic disorder generally does, nonetheless, existing with symptoms.

Typical signs and symptoms of acute nephritic disorder consist of passing much less urine than regular, having blood in the urine, and swelling of the feet or face (edema). Other feasible signs of the nephritic disorder, also depending on the root reason may include:

–   Shortness of breath.

–   Pain in the back and/or sides.

–   Headache.

–   Symptoms associated with the underlying cause, for instance, a breakout or joint pain.

The signs and symptoms of nephritic disorder differ, relying on whether the intense or persistent form of the disorder is being experienced.

Acute pyelonephritis is a common kidney issue in women, particularly those between the ages of 15 and 29. It is quite uneasy; acute pyelonephritis is hardly ever a cause of long term kidney troubles. Some underlying problems can boost the danger of creating severe pyelonephritis.

–   Diabetes.

–   Enlarged prostate/ benign prostatic hyperplasia (BPH).

–   States of immunosuppression, e.g. after obtaining a transplant or in HIV-patients.

–   Pregnancy.

–   Recent severe kidney injury.

Indications Of Nephrotic Syndrome.

The nephrotic disorder is a disorder that indicates that there is an issue with the kidneys, which causes the person shedding significant amounts of healthy protein via their pee. It can affect individuals of any type of age, yet is most commonly the source of kidney troubles in kids, teenagers as well as toddlers. A syndrome is a team of symptoms that commonly take place together as well as create as a result of one more problem.

Signs of severe nephritic disorder include:

- Edema in the face and legs.
- Low manufacturing of urine.
- Blood in the urine.
- Hypertension/high blood pressure.
- Fever.
- Weakness as well as tiredness.
- Loss of appetite.
- Nausea and/or Vomiting.
- Pain in the stomach.
- Malaise (a sensation of general unwellness).

–   The persistent nephritic syndrome usually provides with rather light or perhaps unseen signs, which can consist of:

–   Edema.

–   Hypertension/high blood pressure.

The persistent nephrotic syndrome may lead to kidney failure in its later stages.

In both chronic as well as severe nephritic disorder, the urine will usually include a red cell or components thereof, as the blood cells leakage out of the harmed glomeruli. Urine does not typically consist of red blood cells or the remains of red blood cells.

Indications Of Acute Pyelonephritis

Acute pyelonephritis is an uncomfortable microbial infection of the kidneys which takes place when bacteria enter the urethra, relocate right into the bladder, take a trip up the ureters as well as impact the kidneys. It is typically triggered by the germs Escherichia coli, but can sometimes be triggered by other microorganisms.

One of the unique functions of severe pyelonephritis is lower pain in the back, pain in the side, along the lower ribs or lower abdominal areas, a high temperature of 38 levels Celsius/ 100.4 degrees Fahrenheit or more, chills, nausea and also throwing up. Various other signs of intense pyelonephritis include:

Chronic kidney condition is a common problem, with an approximated 1 in 10 people in the United States having some level of the problem. Chronic kidney disease can take place at any kind of age, yet it is a lot more common in the senior, as well as it is much more typical in women than in guys. In the senior, CKD is usually an outcome of aging instead of an underlying problem.

Indications Of Nephritic Syndrome.

When the kidneys are irritated, the nephritic disorder is the name offered to a collection of indicators and also signs and symptoms that happen. The syndrome is usually the result of a hidden condition such as acute glomerulonephritis, a microbial or viral infection, a systemic problem such as systemic lupus erythematosus, or a hereditary disorder like Alport-Syndrome. A syndrome is a team of symptoms that typically and commonly happen together as well as often establish as a result of an additional condition.

- Pungent or unpleasant-smelling pee.
- Blood in the pee, additionally recognized as hematuria.
- Urinating shateringly or with difficulty.
- Urinating regularly and/or urgently.
- Producing no pee.
- Low blood stress, which can show up as dizziness and/or fatigue.

Some problems incline individuals to chronic kidney disease. These consist of:

Indicators Of Acute Kidney Injury.

Severe kidney injury is a sudden or rapid decrease in kidney function, as well as is thought about a clinical emergency. It happens when there is a direct injury to one or both kidneys, a blockage in an additional condition,, or the ureter creating inadequate blood circulation to the kidneys.

In adults, kidney failure can be created by:

- Low high blood pressure that occurs really instantly and/or is significantly reduced.

- Severe burns.

- Liver failure.

- Severe looseness of the bowels.

- Severe allergic responses.

- Bleeding.

- Coronary artery condition or chronic heart failure.

- Infections.

- Heart assault.

- Dehydration.

Excellent to recognize: People, such as the elderly, the impaired, and youngsters, who are reliant on caretakers for a supply of liquids, go to specific risk of dehydration.

Signs and symptoms of acute kidney failure consist of:

- Poor hunger.

- Nosebleeds.

- Tenderness of the abdomen.

- Swelling in the legs, abdomen, or face.

- Diarrhea.

- Lethargy and/or problem are remaining conscious.

- Breathlessness.

- Passing less pee than typical.

- Rash.

- Nausea, as well as throwing up.

- Asterixis, a sort of spontaneous shaking of the hands.

- Tenderness or pain in the area of the lower ribs.

- Overuse or long-term usage of NSAIDs such as Advil, high dosage pain killers as well as naproxen.

- Smoking.

- A household history of genetic kidney disease.

Various other signs which may look like part of preeclampsia or as preeclampsia proceeds consist of:

- -Oliguria (reduced urine result) of 500ml or less over 24 hrs.
- Nausea and vomiting.
- Confusion or disorientation.
- Blurred vision, various other blind spots, or aesthetic disruptions.
- Being unable to feel the infant action as long as formerly.
- Pain in the top right abdomen, simply below the ribs.
- Headache that can not be alleviated with pain relievers.
- Feeling of great unwellness.
- Edema (swelling) of hands, arms, face, and/or feet.
- Heartburn that can not be eased by antacids.
- Shortness of breath, potentially due to lung edema (excess liquid in the lungs).
- Stroke. This is really rare.

Great to know: If a pregnant person suddenly finds that their watch, rings or armbands no much longer fit their arm or hand, or that their sleeves are all of a sudden tight, they need to look for clinical help right away. Preeclampsia can bring about eclampsia as well as HELLP Syndrome and is taken into consideration a clinical emergency situation.

In youngsters, kidney failure can be triggered by:

- Severe infection.
- Hypotension (reduced high blood pressure).
- Nephritis.
- Severe looseness of the bowels.
- Blood-cell cancer.
- Dehydration.

Indicators Of Kidney Problems During Pregnancy.

Preeclampsia.

Preeclampsia impacts only pregnant ladies after the 20th week of maternity and also deals with soon after the baby is provided. It is by beginning not the main kidney problem; it does involve the kidneys. It is identified by:

- Hypertension.

–   Proteinuria, or healthy protein in the urine.

Various other variables that can enhance the possibility of chronic kidney condition developing are:

Persistent kidney disease may, if not dealt with and managed appropriately, result in acute kidney failure. Signs and symptoms of acute kidney failing consist of:

–   Fever.

–   Diarrhea.

–   Vomiting.

–   Stomach and/or pain in the back.

–   Nosebleeds.

–   Rash.

Indications of later persistent kidney disease.

Chronic kidney condition normally has signs and symptoms only in the middle and also later phases. These consist of:

- Puffiness around the eyes as well as in the face.
- Foggy thinking.
- Nausea.
- Hypertension.
- Fluid retention in the reduced limbs and also feet.
- Poor cravings.
- Pallor.
- Headaches.
- Frequent or urgent urination, specifically in the evening.
- Dry, scratchy skin.
- Fatigue and also a weak point.
- Muscular aches.
- Trouble sleeping.
- A basic sensation of unwellness.

- Weight loss.

- Pulmonary edema.

- Restless legs.

- Neoplasms/Tumor growth.

- Frequent urinary system tract infections.

- Diabetes.

- Glomerulonephritis.

- Multisystem diseases, such as systemic lupus erythematosus.

- Myeloma.

- Hypertension.

- Renal artery stenosis.

- Polycystic kidney disease.

- Blockages to the circulation of urine, from blockages of the urinary system discharge tracts, i.e., the ureter as well as urethra.

Some medicines, such as diuretics, aminoglycoside prescription antibiotics as well as some blood stress tablets, can likewise cause intense kidney failure. Older individuals, as well as people with hidden conditions such as diabetes mellitus, liver condition, or cardiovascular disease, are at increased risk.

In the later phases, various other signs and symptoms might arise, including:

–   Malnutrition.

–   Encephalopathy.

–   Peripheral neuropathy, causing tingling and prickling in the extremities.

–   Pleuritis, inflammation of the cells lining the lungs and chest tooth cavity.

–   Platelet breakdown and irregular blood loss.

–   Pericarditis.

–   Difficulty staying awake.

–   pigmented spots.

–   Decreased sex drive and, in men, impotence.

In serious, persistent kidney disease, missteps, pericarditis, seizures, and also coma might occur. Various other signs and symptoms include anemia and fragile bones due to bone thinning. Signs of anemia include:

- Confusion and also clouded thinking.

- Reduced capacity to work out or complete normal activities.

- Fatigue.

- Impaired immune features causing getting ill extra quickly.

Kidney Stones Or Nephrolithiasis

Kidney stones are generally made up of difficult collections of minerals that form in the renal system. Kidney stones can be extremely agonizing.

Colicky, strong to very strong discomfort, can be found in waves, is the most obvious symptom of kidney stones. The location of the discomfort and where it spreads to gives clues regarding where the stone is currently found in the urinary system. The discomfort of a kidney stone passing through the urinary system is felt unexpectedly and severely in the flank (the side) and spreads out down the groin on the exact same side. Not all stones trigger radiating discomfort. Some stones may not trigger any pain.

Excellent to know: Pain from kidney stones is typically described as agonizing. Kidney discomfort from kidney stones can come and go.

Other symptoms of kidney stones consist of:

- Inability to urinate because of a clog in the ureter.
- Nausea.
- Chills.
- Cloudy and/or bad-smelling urine.
- Hematuria, noticeable blood in the urine.
- Vomiting.
- Fever.
- Painful urination, as well as having to urinate frequently and very urgently or frantically.
- Gravel or stone-like particles in the urine.

10 Signs You May Have Kidney Disease.

If you're at threat for kidney disease due to hypertension, diabetes, a family history of kidney failure, or if you're older than age 60, it's crucial to get tested every year for kidney disease. Make sure to discuss any symptoms you're experiencing to your healthcare professional.

1. You're more worn out, have less energy, or are having difficulty concentrating. A serious reduction in kidney function can cause an accumulation of toxic substances and pollutants in the blood. This can trigger people to feel exhausted, weak and can make it hard to focus. Another problem of kidney disease is anemia, which can cause weak points and fatigue.

2. You're having difficulty sleeping. When the kidneys aren't filtering appropriately, toxic substances remain in the blood rather than leaving the body through the urine. This can make it tough to sleep. There is likewise a link between obesity and chronic kidney disease, and sleep apnea is more typical in those with chronic kidney disease compared with the general population.

3. You have scratchy and dry skin. Healthy kidneys do numerous essential tasks. They eliminate wastes and extra fluid from your body; assistance makes red blood cells, assistance keep bones strong, and work to keep the right quantity of minerals in your blood. Dry and scratchy skin can be an indication of the mineral and bone disease that frequently accompanies advanced kidney disease when the kidneys are no longer able to keep the right balance of minerals and nutrients in your blood.

4. You feel the requirement to urinate more frequently. If you feel the requirement to urinate more frequently, especially during the night, this can be a sign of kidney disease. When the kidney's filters are damaged, it can trigger an increase in the desire to urinate. In some cases this can likewise signify a urinary infection or bigger prostate in males.

5. You see blood in your urine. Healthy kidneys usually keep the blood cells in the body when filtering wastes from the blood to produce urine, but when the kidney's filters have been damaged, these blood cells can start to "leakage" out into the urine. In addition to

signaling kidney disease, blood in the urine can be a sign of tumors, kidney stones, or an infection.

Your urine is foamy. Extreme bubbles in the urine-- particularly those that require you to flush a number of times before they go away-- suggest protein in the urine.

7. You're experiencing consistent puffiness around your eyes. Protein in the urine is an early sign that the kidneys' filters have been damaged, enabling the protein to leakage into the urine. This puffiness around your eyes can be due to the reality that your kidneys are leaking a big amount of protein in the urine, rather than keeping it in the body.

Reduced kidney function can lead to sodium retention, triggering swelling in your ankles and feet. Swelling in the lower extremities can also be a sign of heart disease, liver disease, and persistent leg vein issues.

9. You have a bad hunger. This is a really basic symptom, but a buildup of toxins arising from decreased kidney function can be one of the causes.

Electrolyte imbalances can result from impaired kidney function. Low calcium levels and inadequately controlled phosphorus might contribute to muscle cramping. Kidney stones are generally made up of difficult collections of minerals that form in the renal system. Kidney stones can be extremely agonizing.

Colicky, strong to very strong discomfort, can be found in waves, is the most obvious symptom of kidney stones. The location of the discomfort and where it spreads to gives clues regarding where the stone is currently found in the urinary system. The discomfort of a kidney stone passing through the urinary system is felt unexpectedly and severely in the flank (the side) and spreads out down the groin on the exact same side. Not all stones trigger radiating discomfort. Some stones may not trigger any pain.

Excellent to know: Pain from kidney stones is typically described as agonizing. Kidney discomfort from kidney stones can come and go.

Other symptoms of kidney stones consist of:

- Inability to urinate because of a clog in the ureter.

–	Nausea.

–	Chills.

–	Cloudy and/or bad-smelling urine.

–	Hematuria, noticeable blood in the urine.

–	Vomiting.

–	Fever.

–	Painful urination, as well as having to urinate frequently and very urgently or frantically.

–	Gravel or stone-like particles in the urine.

10 Signs You May Have Kidney Disease.

If you're at threat for kidney disease due to hypertension, diabetes, a family history of kidney failure, or if you're older than age 60, it's crucial to get tested every year for kidney disease. Make sure to discuss any symptoms you're experiencing to your healthcare professional.

1. You're more worn out, have less energy, or are having difficulty concentrating. A serious reduction in kidney function can cause an accumulation of toxic substances and pollutants in the blood. This can trigger people to feel exhausted, weak and can make it hard to focus. Another problem of kidney disease is anemia, which can cause weak points and fatigue.

2. You're having difficulty sleeping. When the kidneys aren't filtering appropriately, toxic substances remain in the blood rather than leaving the body through the urine. This can make it tough to sleep. There is likewise a link between obesity and chronic kidney disease, and sleep apnea is more typical in those with chronic kidney disease compared with the general population.

3. You have scratchy and dry skin. Healthy kidneys do numerous essential tasks. They eliminate wastes and extra fluid from your body; assistance make red blood cells, assistance keep bones strong, and work to keep the right quantity of minerals in your blood. Dry and scratchy skin can be an indication of the mineral and bone disease that frequently accompanies advanced kidney disease when the kidneys are no longer able to keep the right balance of minerals and nutrients in your blood.

4. You feel the requirement to urinate more frequently. If you feel the requirement to urinate more frequently, especially during the night, this can be a sign of kidney disease. When the kidney's filters are damaged, it can trigger an increase in the desire to urinate. In some cases this can likewise signify a urinary infection or bigger prostate in males.

5. You see blood in your urine. Healthy kidneys usually keep the blood cells in the body when filtering wastes from the blood to produce urine, but when the kidney's filters have been damaged, these blood cells can start to "leakage" out into the urine. In addition to

signaling kidney disease, blood in the urine can be a sign of tumors, kidney stones, or an infection.

6. Your urine is foamy. Extreme bubbles in the urine-- particularly those that require you to flush a number of times before they go away-- suggest protein in the urine.

7. You're experiencing consistent puffiness around your eyes. Protein in the urine is an early sign that the kidneys' filters have been damaged, enabling the protein to leakage into the urine. This puffiness around your eyes can be due to the reality that your kidneys are leaking a big amount of protein in the urine, rather than keeping it in the body.

8. Reduced kidney function can lead to sodium retention, triggering swelling in your ankles and feet. Swelling in the lower extremities can also be a sign of heart disease, liver disease, and persistent leg vein issues.

9. You have a bad hunger. This is a really basic symptom, but a buildup of toxins arising from decreased kidney function can be one of the causes.

10. Electrolyte imbalances can result from impaired kidney function. Low calcium levels and inadequately controlled phosphorus might contribute to muscle cramping.

CHRONIC KIDNEY DISEASE

Over 30 million people in the United States are dealing with consistent kidney ailment (CKD).

The term "persistent kidney health problem" suggests lasting damages to the kidneys that can become worse over time. If your kidneys quit working, you will certainly require dialysis or a kidney transplant in order to live.

Persistent kidney condition is a dynamic and also slow loss of kidney features over a period of a number of years. Ultimately, a person will certainly develop permanent kidney failure.

Consistent kidney health problem, additionally called chronic renal failure, persistent kidney disease, or chronic kidney failure, is far more widespread than individuals recognize; it commonly goes undiagnosed as well as undetected up until the health problem is well progressed.

When their kidney function is down to 25 percent of typical, it is not unusual for individuals to understand they have persistent kidney failure just.

As kidney failure developments and also the body organ's feature is significantly damaged, unsafe degrees of waste and also fluid can quickly accumulate in the body. Therapy is targeted at reducing or stopping down the progression of the disease - this is typically done by handling its underlying cause.

Chronic kidney disease (CKD) suggests your kidneys are damaged and also can't filter blood the method they should. The health problem is called "persistent" since the damages to your kidneys happen slowly over a long period of time. CKD can also set off other health issues.

CKD can obtain even worse with time, and eventually the kidneys might stop working entirely, but this is unusual. Persistent kidney disease (CKD) is a lasting problem where the kidneys do not work efficiently.

The last stage of CKD is called end-stage renal disease (ESRD). At this stage, the kidneys are no longer able to eliminate enough wastes as well as excess fluids from the body. Currently, you would need dialysis or a kidney transplant.

Indicators

Persistent kidney failure, rather than intense kidney failing, is a gradually dynamic and slow disease. Also, if one kidney stops operating, the various other can perform normal features. It is not typically until the disease is fairly well innovative and also the problem has actually become severe that symptoms, as well as indicators, are apparent, by which time most of the damage is permanent.

It is essential that people who go to great danger of establishing kidney disease have their kidney works often checked. Early detection can substantially aid avoid serious kidney damage.

The most common indicators of persistent kidney condition consist of:

- anemia.
- blood in pee.
- dark pee.

- reduced psychological understanding.

- decreased urine output.

- edema - swollen feet, hands, as well as ankles (face if edema is serious).

- tiredness (tiredness).

- hypertension (high blood pressure).

- sleeping problems.

- scratchy skin can wind up being regular.

- loss of hunger.

- male failing to get or keep an erection (erectile disorder).

- even more frequent urination, especially throughout the night.

- muscle aches.

- muscular tissue twitches.

- a sick stomach.

- pain on the side or mid to lower back.

- panting (shortness of breath).

- the healthy protein in pee.

- abrupt adjustment in bodyweight.

- unusual migraines.

Stages.

Changes in the GFR price can evaluate just how advanced the kidney condition is. In the UK, and several various other countries, kidney disease stages are classified as complies with:

Phase 1 - GFR price is normal. Proof of kidney disease has been discovered.

Stage 2 - GFR rate is reduced than 90 milliliters, as well as evidence of kidney health problem, has actually been spotted.

Phase 3 - GFR price is less than 60 milliliters, regardless of whether proof of kidney disease has, in fact been discovered.

Phase 4 - GRF price is less than 30 milliliters, no matter whether proof of kidney health problem has actually been determined.

Stage 5 - GFR price is reduced than 15 milliliters. Renal failure has actually taken place.

Most of the customers with persistent kidney disease hardly ever growth beyond Stage 2. It is essential for kidney disease to be identified as well as managed early for significant damage to be stopped.

Clients with diabetes mellitus should have a yearly test, which measures microalbuminuria (little quantities of healthy protein) in the urine. This examination can detect very early diabetic person nephropathy (very early kidney damage connected to diabetic issues).

Treatment.

There is no present solution for persistent kidney disease. Some therapies can aid in regulating the signs and also signs, lessen the risk of problems, and slow down the progression of the ailment.

People with persistent kidney disease typically require to take a wide variety of medications. Treatments include:

Anemia treatment.

Hemoglobin is the substance in red cells that brings essential oxygen around the body. If hemoglobin levels are low, the person has anemia.

Some kidney disease customers with anemia will need blood transfusions. A client with kidney disease will normally need to take iron supplements, either in the type of day-to-day ferrous sulfate tablet computers or occasionally in the kind of shots.

Phosphate equilibrium.

Individuals with kidney conditions could not be able to remove phosphate from their bodies properly. People will certainly be recommended to minimize their nutritional phosphate consumption - this generally suggests lowering consumption of milk products, red meat, eggs, and fish.

Hypertension.

Hypertension is a common problem for patients with consistent kidney disease. It is extremely vital to bring high blood stress to guard the kidneys, and also consequently decrease the growth of the disease.

Skin itching.

Antihistamines, such as chlorphenamine, might aid in alleviating indicators of itching.

Anti-sickness drugs.

If toxic materials develop in the body because the kidneys do not function properly, customers may feel unwell (a sick stomach) — medications such as cyclizine or metoclopramide assistance simplicity disease.

NSAIDs (nonsteroidal anti-inflammatory medicines).

NSAIDs, such as pain killers or ibuprofen, need to be stayed clear of and simply taken if a doctor suggests them.

End-stage treatment.

When the kidneys are functioning at much less than 10-15 percent of typical ability, this is. Procedures consumed previously - diet regimen, medicines, and also therapies managing underlying causes - are no much longer sufficient. The kidneys of clients with end-stage kidney disease cannot stay up to a day with the waste and liquid elimination process on their own - the individual will certainly call for dialysis or a kidney transplant in order to survive.

Because they carry the risk of possibly severe issues, a lot of physicians will certainly attempt to postpone the requirement for dialysis or a kidney transplant for as long as possible.

Kidney dialysis.

This is the elimination of waste items as well as severe liquids from the blood when the kidneys can avoid doing the job effectively anymore. Dialysis has some severe risks, including infection.

There are 2 primary kinds of kidney dialysis. Each type additionally has subtypes. The 2 major types are:

Hemodialysis: Blood is drained of the client's body and undergoes a dialyzer (a synthetic kidney). The client experiences hemodialysis about three times once a week. Each session lasts for at least 3 hrs.

Professionals now recognize that even more frequent sessions lead to a much better lifestyle for the person. However, contemporary home-use dialysis makers are making this even more regular use hemodialysis feasible.

Peritoneal dialysis: The blood is a filtering system in the client's very own abdominal area, in the peritoneal tooth cavity which consists of a substantial network of little blood vessels. A catheter is implanted right into the abdomen, into which a dialysis solution is infused and also drained out for as long as is called to eliminate waste and excess fluid.

Kidney transplant.

A kidney transplant is a much better option than dialysis for customers that have nothing else conditions apart from kidney failure. However, candidates for kidney transplant will certainly have to go with dialysis till they get a new kidney.

The kidney contributor, as well as recipient, must have the precise very same blood group, cell-surface healthy proteins, and also antibodies in order to lower the danger of rejection of the brand-new kidney. Siblings or incredibly close family members are normally the best kinds of benefactors. If a living donor is not possible, the search will start for a body contributor (dead individual).

Diet

Adhering to a suitable diet plan is essential for efficient kidney failing treatment. Restricting the amount of protein in the diet regimen could assist reduce the growth of the ailment.

Diet regimen may similarly help soothe symptoms of queasiness.

Salt consumption should be thoroughly controlled to take care of hypertension. Potassium and phosphorus use, with time, could likewise require to be restricted.

Vitamin D.

Patients with kidney health problems typically have low levels of vitamin D. Vitamin D is required for healthy bones. The vitamin D we obtain from the sun or food has actually to be caused by the kidneys before the body can utilize it. People might be provided alfacalcidol or calcitriol.

Fluid retention.

Individuals with consistent kidney ailments need to be careful with their liquid usage. A lot of clients will certainly be asked to restrict their fluid consumption. The customer is a lot much more vulnerable to fluid accumulation if the kidneys do not work correctly.

Reasons.

Kidneys execute the complex system of filtering systems in our bodies - excess waste, and liquid products are eliminated from the blood and also eliminated from the body.

Essentially, kidneys can do away with many waste items that our body creates. If the blood circulation to the kidneys is impacted, they are not functioning properly as a result of the truth that of damages or ailment, or if pee outflow is obstructed, problems can take place.

Generally, progressive kidney damage is the result of a chronic disease (a resilient ailment), such as:

- Diabetes - relentless kidney disease is linked to diabetic issues kinds 1 and 2. Excess sugar (sugar) can accumulate in the blood if the customer's diabetes mellitus is not well managed. Kidney condition is not regular throughout the first 10 years of diabetes; it extra typically takes place 15-25 years after diagnosis of diabetes.

- Hypertension (hypertension) - hypertension can harm the glomeruli - components of the kidney related to filtering waste things.

- Obstructed urine blood circulation - if urine flow is obstructed, it can support the kidney from the bladder (vesicoureteral reflux). Blocked pee blood circulation enhances pressure on the kidneys as well as deteriorates their features. Possible reasons consist of a larger prostate, kidney rocks, or growth.

Kidney ailment - including polycystic kidney glomerulonephritis, condition, or pyelonephritis.

Kidney artery stenosis - the kidney artery tightens or is obstructed prior to it enters the kidney.

Certain toxic substances - including fuels, solvents (such as carbon tetrachloride), as well as lead (and also lead-based paint, pipelines, as well as soldering materials). Even some type of jewelry has impurities, which can trigger relentless kidney failing.

Fetal developing issue - if the kidneys do not create correctly in the unborn youngster while it is establishing in the womb.

Systemic lupus erythematosus - an autoimmune ailment. The body's own body's immune system assaults the kidneys as though they were international tissue.

Malaria and yellow fever - understood to activate damaged kidney function.

Some medications - overuse of, for example, NSAIDs (non-steroidal anti-inflammatory medications), such as pain killers or Advil.

Illegal chemical abuse - such as heroin or drug.

Injury - a sharp impact or physical injury to the kidney(s).

Danger elements.

The following conditions or conditions are linked to a greater risk of establishing kidney disease:

- a household background of kidney disease.

- age - chronic kidney disease is even more usual among individuals over 60.

- atherosclerosis.

- bladder blockage.

- persistent glomerulonephritis.

- hereditary kidney disease (kidney condition which exists at birth).

- diabetes mellitus - among the most usual threat facets.

- hypertension.

- lupus erythematosus.

- too much exposure to some toxic substances.

- sickle cell disease.

- some medications.

Clinical medical diagnosis.

A physician will certainly inspect for indications and ask the client about indications. The following examinations may similarly be purchased:

- Blood examination - a blood test might be purchased to determine whether waste compounds are being properly strained. If degrees of urea, as well as creatinine, are constantly high, the medical expert will certainly most likely identify end-stage kidney disease.

- Urine test - a urine test helps discover whether there is either blood or healthy protein in the urine.

- Kidney scans - kidney scans could contain a magnetic resonance imaging (MRI) scan, computed tomography (CT) check, or an ultrasound check. The objective is to recognize whether there is any kind of clogs in the urine circulation. These scans can additionally disclose the shapes and size of the kidneys - in sophisticated phases of kidney disease the kidneys are smaller sized and have an uneven form.

- Kidney biopsy - a little sample of kidney tissue is attracted out and taken an appearance at for cell damages. Evaluation of kidney tissue makes it much simpler to make an accurate diagnosis of kidney disease.

- Chest X-ray - the purpose below is to seek lung edema (fluid retained in the lungs).

- Glomerular purification price (GFR) - GFR is a test that determines the glomerular purification rate - it compares the degrees of waste items in the customer's blood and also pee. GFR tips the variety of milliliters of waste the kidneys can filter per minute. The kidneys of healthy and balanced individuals can commonly filter over 90 ml per min.

Troubles

If chronic kidney disease progresses to kidney failure, the complying with difficulties are possible:

- anemia.
- main nerve system damages.
- dry skin or skin color adjustments.
- fluid retention.

–   hyperkalemia, when blood potassium levels enhance, potentially causing heart damages.

–   sleeping conditions.

–   lower libido.

–   man erectile dysfunction.

–   osteomalacia, when bones come to be weak and break quickly.

–   pericarditis, when the sac-like membrane around the heart becomes irritated.

–   tummy abscess.

–   weak body immune system.

Avoidance.

Handling the chronic problem.

Some conditions boost the danger of persistent kidney disease (such as diabetes test Mellitus). Managing the problem can significantly decrease the possibility of establishing kidney failing. Individuals should follow their medical professional's directions, advice, and recommendations.

Diet.

A healthy and balanced diet plan consisting of lots of fruits and also veggies, whole grains, and lean meats or fish will certainly aid in maintaining high blood stress down.

Exercise.

Routine exercise is suitable for maintaining healthy hypertension degrees; it also aids chronic control conditions such as diabetes as well as heart trouble. Individuals should contact a physician that an exercise program is matched to their weight, age, and health.

Stopping details substances.

Containing abusing alcohol and medicines. Protect against long-lasting straight exposure to hefty metals, such as lead. Protect against lasting direct exposure to gas, solvents, and also other unsafe chemicals.

KIDNEY STONES

When your pee has high degrees of these salts and also minerals, you can form stones. If the stone reaches the bladder, it can be lost awareness of the body in pee. If the rock winds up being lodged in the ureter, it obstructs the pee flow from that kidney as well as triggers discomfort.

The Kidneys And Urinary System

The kidneys are fist-sized body organs that manage the body's fluid and also chemical degrees. Healthy and balanced kidneys tidy waste from the blood as well as remove it in the pee.

The kidneys make urine from water and also your body's waste. The urine after that takes a trip down the ureters into the bladder, where it is maintained.

Kidney stones develop in the kidney. It is called a ureteral rock if a stone gets and also leaves the kidney stuck in the ureter.

What Are Kidney Stones Made Of?

Kidney stones come in several kinds and shades. How you treat them and also stop new rocks from developing depends upon what sort of stone you have.

Calcium stones (80 percent of stones).

Calcium rocks are the most typical kind of kidney stone. Also, with normal amounts of calcium in the pee, calcium stones might create for various other aspects.

Uric acid stones (5-10 percent of rocks).

Uric acid is a waste item that originates from chemical alterations in the body. Uric acid crystals do not dissolve well in acidic pee and also rather will form a uric acid rock. Having acidic pee could originate from:

- Being overweight.
- Chronic looseness of the bowels.
- Type 2 diabetes (high blood glucose degree).
- Gout.

– A diet regimen that is high in healthy animal protein and also low in veggies as well as fruits.

Struvite/infection rocks (10 percent of stones).

Struvite rocks are not the usual kind of stone. Magnesium ammonium phosphate (struvite) rocks create in alkaline urine.

Individuals who get persistent UTIs, such as those with long-term tubes in their bladders or kidneys, or individuals with bad bladder clearing due to neurologic conditions (paralysis, multiple sclerosis, and also spina bifida) are at the best threat for establishing these rocks.

Cystine stones (less than 1 percent of stones).

When high quantities of cystine remain in the pee, it causes stones to develop. Cystine stones frequently begin to develop in young people.

Signs And Symptoms.

When a stone leaves the kidney, it travels to the bladder via the ureter. When the stone blocks the circulation of pee out of the kidney, it can trigger the kidney to swell (hydronephrosis), frequently activating a great deal of pain.

Usual signs of kidney stones are:

Some ladies state the pain is also worse than childbirth labor pains. It can go as well as come as the body tries to obtain rid of the rock.

- A sensation of extreme need to urinate.

- Urinating more regularly or a burning feeling throughout urination.

- Urine that is dark or red because of blood. In some cases, urine has just percentages of red cells that can't be seen with the nude eye.

- Nausea and also throwing up.

- For males, you may feel discomfort at the idea of the penis.

Reasons.

Reduced Urine Volume.

A significant danger aspect for kidney rocks is consistent low urine volume. Reduced urine volume might stem from dehydration (loss of body fluids) from a difficult workout, living or working in a hot place, or otherwise drinking sufficient liquids. When urine volume is reduced, pee is dark and also focused in the shade. Focused pee recommends there is less fluid to keep salts liquified. Raising fluid consumption will certainly thin down the salts in your urine. By doing this, you may reduce your danger of rocks creating.

Grownups that form stones should certainly drink sufficient fluid to make at the very least 2.5 liters (2/3 gallons) of pee each day. Typically, this will certainly take around 3 liters (100 ounces) of liquid consumption every day. While water is more than likely the very best fluid to consume, what matters most is getting adequate fluid.

Diet.

One of the lot more common root causes of calcium kidney stones is high degrees of calcium in the pee. Reducing the amount of calcium in your diet regimen rarely quits rocks from creating. Research studies have revealed that limiting nutritional calcium can be poor for bone health and might increase kidney stone risk.

Decreasing salt in the diet plan reduces pee calcium, making it less more than likely for calcium rocks to create. Because oxalate belongs to one of the most usual types of kidney stones (calcium oxalate), consuming foods plentiful in oxalate can raise your risk of developing these rocks.

A diet plan high in animal protein, such as beef, pork, fish, and chicken, can raise the acid levels in the body and in the urine. High acid levels make it easier for calcium oxalate and uric acid stones to form. The breakdown of meat into uric acid also raises the possibility that both calcium and uric acid stones will form.

Digestive tract Conditions

Specific bowel problems that create diarrhea (such as Crohn's Disease or ulcerative colitis) or surgical treatments (such as stomach bypass surgical treatment) can elevate the threat of developing calcium oxalate kidney stones. Both low pee quantity and high degrees of urine oxalate can assist in creating calcium oxalate kidney stone formation.

Weight issues

Weight issues are a threat aspect of rocks. Weight issues might alter the acid levels in the pee, leading to stone development.

Clinical problems

Some medical problems have actually an increased danger of kidney rocks. Unusual growth of several of the parathyroid glands, which manage calcium metabolic process, can cause high calcium levels in the blood as well as urine. This can bring about kidney rocks. Another problem called distal renal tubular acidosis, in which there is acid accumulation in the body, can elevate the risk of calcium phosphate kidney rocks.

Some uncommon, gotten conditions can likewise make details sorts of stones a lot more than likely. Examples include cystinuria, which is excessive of the amino acid cystine in the pee, and also key hyperoxaluria, in which the liver makes as well much oxalate.

Medication

Some medicines, as well as calcium and also vitamin C supplements, may raise your threat of creating rocks. Make particular to inform your health care provider all the supplements and also drugs you take, as these can affect your threat of rock development. Do not quit taking any one of these unless your health care provider informs you to do so.

Family members History

The opportunity of having kidney stones is a lot higher if you have a house history of stones, such as a parent or brother or sister.

Diagnosis

" Silent" kidney rocks, those that cause no signs, are often uncovered when an X-ray is taken throughout a wellness assessment. Various other individuals have their rocks identified when sudden pain happens while the stone is passing, as well as medical interest is needed.

When a person has blood in the pee (hematuria) or sudden abdominal or side discomfort, tests like a ct or an ultrasound check could identify a stone. These imaging tests tell the health and wellness treatment company exactly how large the rock is and where it exists.

When a rock is suspected, a CT scan is commonly made use of in the ER. Because of the fact that it can make a precise as well as quick clinical diagnosis, it is utilized.

Treatment

Treatment relies on the kind of rock, how poor it is as well as the length of time you have actually had signs and symptoms. There are various treatments to pick from. It is essential to speak to your health care company about what is ideal for you.

Wait for the rock to pass by itself

Often you can simply await the stone to pass. Smaller sized rocks are much more likely than bigger stones to hand down their very own.

Waiting as long as 4 to 6 weeks for the stone to pass is secure as long as the pain is manageable, there are no signs of infection, the kidney is not entirely blocked, and also the rock is little sufficient that it is likely to pass. While waiting for the stone to pass, you should drink normal quantities of water. You might require pain drugs when there is pain.

Drug

Particular medicines have actually been revealed to boost the opportunity that a stone will certainly pass. Tamsulosin (Flomax) loosens up the ureter, making it much less complicated for the rock to pass.

Surgical procedure

Surgical treatment could be required to eliminate a rock from the ureter or kidney if:

The stone quits working to pass.

The pain is unnecessary to wait on the rock to pass.

The stone is influencing kidney function. If they are not creating discomfort or infection, little stones in the kidney might be left alone.

Kidney rocks need to be removed by surgical therapy if they cause copied infections in the pee or as a result of the fact that they are blocking the blood circulation of pee from the kidney. Today, surgery generally includes little or no incisions (cuts), small pain, and also marginal pause job.

Surgical treatments to eliminate rocks in the ureters or kidneys are:

Shock wave lithotripsy (SWL).

Shock waves are concentrated on the rock using X-rays or ultrasound to establish the stone. The repetitive shooting of shock waves on the stone usually causes the rock to break into small items.

Because of feasible pain induced by the shock waves and also the requirement to manage to breathe throughout the therapy, some form of anesthesia is frequently needed. SWL does not work well on hard stones, such as cystine, some kinds of calcium oxalate and also calcium phosphate stones, or really big rocks.

You might likewise be offered a strainer to accumulate the stone items as they pass. These items will be sent to the lab to be evaluated.

Lots of rock pieces pass painlessly. Larger items might obtain stuck in the ureter, causing pain as well as requiring other removal therapies.

Ureteroscopy (URS).

Ureteroscopy (URS) is utilized to treat stones in the kidney and also ureter. Functional telescopes are made use of to deal with stones in the upper ureter as well as the kidney.

The ureteroscope lets the urologist see the stone without making an incision (cuts). General anesthetic keeps you comfy throughout the URS therapy. As soon as the urologist sees the stone with the ureteroscope, a little, basket-like device grabs smaller rocks as well as removes them. If a rock is too huge to eliminate unscathed, it can be gotten into smaller sized pieces with a laser or various other stone-breaking tools.

When the rock has actually been eliminated whole or in pieces, the medical care company may place a short-lived stint in the ureter. A stent is a tiny, stiff plastic tube that aids hold the ureter open so that urine can drain pipes from the kidney right into the bladder. Unlike a catheter or PCNL drain tube, this tube is completely within the body and also does not require an exterior bag to collect pee.

It is extremely vital that the stent is eliminated when your healthcare supplier tells you. Leaving the stent in for a long period of time can activate an infection as well as loss of kidney feature.

Percutaneous nephrolithotomy (PCNL).

Percutaneous Lithotripsy (PCNL) is the extremely finest treatment for big stones in the kidney. General anesthesia is required to do a PCNL. PCNL entails making a half-inch cut (cut) in the back or side, simply large enough to permit a rigid telescope (nephroscope) to be gone into the hollow center component of the kidney where the stone lies.

An instrument undergone the nephroscope separates the stone and also suctions out the items. The ability to suction pieces makes PCNL the best therapy alternative for large rocks.

After the PCNL, a tube is generally left in the kidney to drain pee right into a bag beyond the body. This will make it possible for water drainage of urine as well as stop any blood loss. Tv is left in overnight or for a couple of days. You may need to remain in the health care center overnight hereafter operation.

Your urologist may select to do X-rays while you are still in the university hospital to see if any type of rock items remain. As soon as again to remove them if there are any type of, your urologist could want to look back into the kidney with a telescope. You can begin common activities after regarding one-to-two weeks.

Various other medical therapy.

Another kidney surgical procedure is rarely made use of to remove rocks. Open, laparoscopic or robotic medical therapy might be used simply if all other less invasive treatments fall short.

TREATMENT AND PREVENTION

Kidney conditions are quiet killers. They might cause modern loss of kidney function resulting in kidney failure and also inevitably demand dialysis or kidney transplant to suffer life. Since of the high expense and also potential problems of absence of availability in establishing countries, only 5 -10% of patients with kidney failure are privileged adequate to obtain clear-cut therapy choices such as dialysis and also kidney hair transplant, while the rest pass away without getting any conclusive treatment. Chronic kidney disease (CKD) is extremely typical and also has no remedy, so avoidance is the only choice. Early discovery and therapy can usually maintain CKD from worsening, and also can protect against or postpone the requirement for definitive therapy.

Kidney Failure And Its Treatment

Kidney failure additionally called renal failure. It is a critical disease which can have a primary impact on life, and also can become dangerous. However, it can be cured.

Kidney failure is additionally related to a rise in the amount of water in the body, which can impact the swelling of the cells. Healthy and balanced kidneys wash your blood by removing excess fluid, minerals, and wastes. They make hormonal agents that safeguard your bones strong as well as your blood well also. If the organs are damaged, they don't run properly.

This is called kidney failure. It is a state in which the kidneys fail to function completely.

Kidney failure can generally be divided into 2 kinds: severe kidney failing as well as persistent kidney disease. Acute failure is the hasty loss of the capacity of the kidneys to remove waste as well as intentional urine without shedding electrolytes.

The kind of kidney failing (persistent vs. acute) is developed by the trend in the serum creatinine. Various other things that potentially will help to distinguish intensely and also persistent kidney disease include the visibility of anemia and also the kidney dimension on ultrasound. Enduring, i.e. chronic, kidney disease, commonly causes anemia and little kidney size.

At least, there are three choices when treating kidney failure:

1. Hemodialysis

2. Peritoneal dialysis

3. Kidney transplant

Every therapy has advantages as well as disadvantages. Regardless of which treatment you select, you'll have to make some modifications in your life, consisting of how you eat and also prepare your activities. Yet with the help of a doctor, family members, and good friends, the majority people with kidney failure can run completely satisfied as well as energetic lives.

For a suitable individual at the ideal time, a transplant is the finest treatment for kidney failure. If it operates effectively the person will be total without dialysis. Many people with kidney failure are proper for a transplant.

Kidney failure can happen quickly (days) or more unhurriedly (months or years). A lot of conditions can produce kidneys to fail, making up diabetes and high blood pressure. Lots of individuals with chronic kidney failing necessitate take medications, and also lots of demand dialysis.

Kidney Failure Treatment Without Dialysis

Kidney failing might set in as a result of several possible reasons consisting of long term use of over-the-counter and also prescription medications, health problems, exposure to chemicals over an extended period of time. Symptoms of kidney failure include vomiting, queasiness, persistent back troubles, and blood or protein in pee. Individuals can go with expensive choices like transplant or dialysis or for kidney failure therapy without dialysis

Techniques of kidney failing treatment without dialysis.

Right here are a couple of ways of dealing with kidney failure without choosing dialysis or transplant:

Consist of such food products in your diet plan that can be absorbed easily by the body. Stay clear of foodstuff, which puts tension on the kidneys for obtaining digested.

Specific natural herbs aid in detoxification of kidneys and boost their health and wellness. Before beginning usage of any one of over such herbs, do not fail to remember consulting your medical professional, particularly if you are taking prescription medicines.

Hoelen is one more herb that can confirm to be useful for kidney clients. Three to six grams of the dried out herb will certainly be excellent sufficient for preventing buildup of lesions in the kidney.

Cranberries: Urinary tract infections can be protected against by eating cranberry juice. Pure, bitter cranberry juice ought to be picked instead of cranberry juice mixed drink as the latter has high sugar levels.

4. Flaxseed: A whole lot has actually been claimed and blogged about exactly how efficiently flaxseed sustains kidney functions. In fact, flaxseed is abundant in omega-3 fatty acids as well as alpha-linolenic acid, which offers enough quantity of assistance to the kidneys. These 2 substances are fairly efficient in stopping inflammation and obstructing of arteries.

Marshmallow: Kidney individuals should seriously consider consuming alcohol marshmallows for increasing kidney features. Drinking one quart of marshmallow daily is rather efficient in cleaning the kidneys. This technique can benefit people of kidney stones.

Kidney failure people need to prevent specific food products. Such food things consist of those with high salt web content. Oregano, basil, or parsley can be made use of to substitute salt for flavoring the food. Salad dressings, canned foods, barbeque sauce, bacon and also various other food items having high salt web content must be avoided.

As shown by the above lines, one can conquer kidney failure with specific easy remedies. Kidney failing treatment without dialysis is quite feasible. All you require is some expertise and also lots of specialist suggestions.

How To Prevent Kidney Failure

For those who experience kidney disease, you will certainly understand just how essential it is to protect against kidney failing Kidney condition can be both long-term and also short-lived. This can be called severe kidney failure/acute renal failure or persistent kidney failure.

The difference between acute as well as chronic renal failure.

With acute kidney failure, the function of the kidneys is swiftly lost and can happen from numerous anxieties on the body, a lot of which are associated with diet plan. Others are indirectly associated with diet, being brought on by another condition or ailment. There are several categories of intense kidney disease as well as is popularized into the complying with groups:

Usual Pre-renal Causes of Kidney Disease

- dehydration from excess liquid loss (diarrhea, influenza, gastroenteritis, sweating).

- dehydration from the absence of fluid intake.

- hypovolemia from excess blood loss.

- obstruction of kidney arteries, as well as veins, are creating irregular blood circulation.

- pain reliever, various other medication as well as excess sodium/potassium/protein.

Usual Post-renal Causes of Renal Failure.

- Having any type of constraint in the bladder can create back-flow to the kidneys. This can create a collection of occasions, from infection to totally damaging the kidneys due to the excess pressure.

- Blockages, cysts, tumors in the abdominal area can create obstructions around the ureters.

- Other age-relevant obstructions, consisting of cancers and also other tumors around the bladder.

–   Having kidney rocks does not directly influence kidney failure but does boost the risk; however, having a great deal of added strain on the kidneys.

Typical Causes of Kidney Damage.

–   Toxic Medications are discovered in specific prescription antibiotics, ibuprofen, some anti-inflammatory medicines, iodine and also radiology medications.

–   Sepsis can happen if the body's body immune system is fighting infection. This can create the kidneys to close down because of this.

–   Muscle malfunction can cause muscle mass fibers, which are damaged to clog filtration of the kidneys. This can generally get on established by serious injury as well as burns to the body.

–   inflammation of the kidney filtering system - the glomeruli.

Typical Causes of Chronic Kidney Failure.

–   Many problems noted above can cause chronic kidney failure.

- continuous hypertension.

- people are suffering diabetes.

- persistent glomerulonephritis.

- kidney stones.

- prostate disease or prostate cancer.

- reflux nephropathy.

- polycystic problems.

HOW TO CURE KIDNEY DISEASE NATURALLY

If you've been diagnosed with Chronic Kidney Disease lately, you probably have a lot of unanswered concerns in your mind. In the list of "ifs, buts, what're whys and just how's" one of the most vital inquiries you require to deal with is - What next?

Kidney disease treatments include prescription drugs, dialysis as well as transplant. All the treatment measures stated are pharmaceutical approaches and also not natural condition therapies.

There is a lot of individuals on the planet today that experience from kidney condition as well as numerous really feel that there is no expect recuperation or even a somewhat regular lifestyle. This might have been real a few years earlier, but today there are people available searching for different techniques and useful suggestions for dealing with all different kinds of kidney diseases.

This section loses light on all-natural therapies for renal issues.

Kidney disease natural treatments include nutritional changes, usage of the natural herb, and also important oils.

1 Diet:

Diet regimen is a vital component of chronic kidney disease therapy. A lot of dietitians advise preventing foods abundant in salt. This includes salty snacks like crackers, tinned vegetables, as well as canned soups, processed cheeses, as well as meats and icy dinners. Eat lower potassium foods. Fruits such as apples, grapes, watermelons, and also strawberries and vegetables such as cabbages and environment-friendly beans are instances of reduced potassium foods. You need to stay clear of foods such as bananas, tomatoes, oranges, potatoes as well as spinach. Protein is required for muscle growth and also toughness. However, it is not a valuable option for renal troubles. A dietician will certainly make referrals of the maximum quantity of grams of proteins you ought to eat daily.

2 Home Remedies:

Apple Cider Vinegar, Baking soft drink, and corn silk are natural substances to recover kidney infections. A pinch of cooking soft drink contributed to a glass of water restores the acid-base equilibrium of pee. You need to drink bitter cranberry juice every day. It prevents the facility of germs by making the pee acidic. Juniper berries achieve the very same impact. An additional all-natural remedy is to eat one husk of garlic every day. Utilize a home heating pad to eliminate discomfort triggered by kidney conditions.

3 Herbal Treatments:

A variety of natural herbs, a lot of obtained from Chinese herbal remedies, have actually aided solve or at least offer remedy for kidney issues. Numerous amongst these are back by scientific researches. Herbs operate in different ways. Some are anti-inflammatory and also anti-bacterial representatives, while certain herbs help the kidneys eliminate waste products. Kidney advantageous herbs are Dandelion root and also Lei Gong Teng. Organic therapies require details precautions. One needs to take them in the dose and also kindly suggested by a professional of natural medicine. You need likewise to keep the nephrologist managing your case informed on making use of such natural treatments.

4 Preventive Measures

Avoidance is constantly much better than treatment. Follow these ideas to avoid the start of a kidney condition or infection.

- You can drink alcohol, however, in moderation.

- Over-the-counter and also prescription drugs are made use of to dealt with health and wellness conditions. Long term usage starts kidney damage. Drugs need to be absorbed the prescribed way just.

- Quit cigarette smoking. It is the most effective health choice you can make, not only for your kidneys yet likewise for your lungs.

- Obesity, like diabetes and hypertension, increases health complications. Keep healthy and balanced weight by consuming right and also exercising regularly.

Kidney conditions need not be taken gently. A very early medical diagnosis and suitable kidney disease therapy measures will boost feature and increase the top quality of your life.

Calcium And Kidney Stones - How To Pass Kidney Stones Naturally

Calcium, as well as kidney rocks, go with each other. Actually, about 9 in every 10 kidney stones are made up of calcium. This is fantastic information because calcium kidney rocks are the most basic to treat normally as well as they can actually be dissolved.

In this section, you will certainly learn exactly how to pass them normally with straightforward treatments and common foods.

Consume Plenty of Water for Kidney Stones

I am guessing that you have already tried consuming a lot of water for treating you your condition. You ought to quickly begin doing this if you have not. Water is very important for the kidneys to operate effectively.

Actually, many calcium rocks are the result of not consuming alcohol sufficient water to purge the calcium (called dehydration). But besides drinking a lot of water, there are likewise other things that you can do today.

Pass Calcium Kidney Stones Naturally

1. Consume a minimum of 100 ounces of water the whole day. You should drink at the very least 1 mug for each hour you are awake.

2. Consuming lemon day-to-day (include in water) can also benefit the kidneys by assisting the rocks dissolve. The citric acid (in lemons) can be valuable for dissolving calcium deposits in the kidneys.

3. Exercise daily to change the stones and also assist them to pass.

4. Eating a lot of fruits, veggies, entire grains, and bran can give fiber also to assist purge the kidneys. You need to eat at least 7 servings of fruits or veggies daily.

5. Resting at the very least 8 hours an evening will also aid.

6. Some studies show that taking a magnesium supplement at 300 to 350 mg daily can additionally be advantageous.

7. You should additionally avoid eating a lot of sugar, which has been linked with a higher threat of this disease.

8. Phosphoric acid is, without a doubt the greatest dissolvent for passing calcium rocks. Learn what beverages have this crucial acid.

HOW TO AVOID DIALYSIS THROUGH DRUG TREATMENTS

It's terrifying to be diagnosed with persistent kidney disease (CKD) if you find out in the very early stages of the disease, there are actions you can take to prolong kidney feature. Opportunities are great; you can still appreciate a healthful top quality of life with kidney condition if you function closely with your medical professional.

Following health techniques, remaining on the work as well as remaining to take pleasure in social tasks are methods a person can feel in control of their condition. Along with doing everything physically and clinically possible to extend kidney features, having a job with wellness insurance policy provides security that income, as well as wellness advantages, will certainly be offered.

Dialysis

Dialysis is a therapy for kidney failure. There are two sorts of dialysis: hemodialysis as well as peritoneal dialysis. Hemodialysis makes use of a machine to cleanse your blood. This sort of dialysis can be done at a dialysis center or in a tidy area in your home. Hemodialysis that is performed in a dialysis center is called in-center hemodialysis, as well as it is one of the most common treatments for kidney failure. Peritoneal dialysis uses the lining of your abdomen (stubborn belly area), called your abdominal muscle, as a filter to clean your blood. This sort of dialysis can be done anywhere that is completely dry and also tidy.

Dialysis utilizes devices to clean your blood as well as do a few of the jobs (around 10%) that healthy and balanced kidneys do. Dialysis can aid with signs brought on by kidney failure; however if you have various other medical conditions, e.g. stroke, Parkinson's disease, peripheral vascular condition, frailty, or dementia, dialysis will not assist with the signs and symptoms that they create, as well as might also make them worse. Dialysis does not stop your kidney function wearing away better; as a matter of fact, it can often make it worsen quicker.

Dialysis can be a troublesome treatment and might minimize high quality of life, specifically in patients with various other medical conditions. Dialysis therapy does not constantly prolong life in people with other clinical conditions; even if it does, a lot of the additional days of life obtained might be spent in health center.

After taking these and also other variables into consideration, some people pick not to begin dialysis; however instead select energetic encouraging treatment (in some cases referred to as traditional, optimal traditional or responsive care).

There are many reasons for CKD; there are certain referrals that, when complied with, can aid a person in delay kidney failure, which leads to dialysis or kidney transplant.

The two primary reasons for CKD in Americans are diabetes and high blood pressure. This disease should be controlled-- or prevented-- to assist extend kidney function.

Diabetes and also extending kidney feature

Diabetics require to maintain their blood sugar level in an acceptable variety as well as take all physician-prescribed medicines. Furthermore, the hemoglobin A1c must be maintained listed below 6.5 percent, and also kidney function tests need to be done at the very least yearly. Studies have shown that specific hypertension medications can protect the kidneys of individuals with diabetic issues, also if they have typical high blood pressure.

High blood pressure and prolonging kidney features.

Individuals with hypertension, also understood as hypertension, should take their blood stress medication as directed by their physician. The National Heart, Lung, and also Blood Institute recommends that blood pressure remains in control at 125/75 or lower for those with kidney troubles, which are not diabetic persons, or 130/85 or lower for those with diabetes.

Various other disease that causes kidney damage

Various other disease that can damage kidneys includes IgA nephropathy, lupus as well as glomerulonephritis. With these diseases the body's immune system overacts, and also inflammation happens in the kidneys. To reduce the disease process, a medical professional might recommend steroids and other drugs.

CKD might likewise be prompted by infections, obstructions, and medications that damage the kidneys. Infections can often be cleared up with antibiotics. Obstructions might be eliminated with surgical procedures or other treatments. Particular medicines, such as prescription and also non-prescription painkillers, some anti-biotics as well as comparison dye (utilized in medical screening) may have negative effects on the kidneys. A client needs to talk their physicians that they have CKD and also supply a checklist of all the medications they are taking, consisting of over-the-counter drugs, to stop further kidney damage.

Actions to prolong kidney function

No matter exactly how an individual creates CKD, there are actions an individual can take to extend kidney features. Cigarette smoking creates quicker progression of kidney condition. As a result, it's advised that those with kidney disease stop smoking. Lots of doctors believe that also avoiding much protein as well as phosphorus in the diet might additionally slow the development of kidney disease.

Remember, your kidney problem is special. You can speak with your medical professional and work with your wellness treatment group for personalized tips on how to extend your kidney function. A constant and also open dialog will certainly create the most effective results. As discussing your medical condition, talk to your medical professional about your sensations as well as ask for suggestions on exactly how to speak with your household about CKD. Your health care group wishes to assist keep you healthy both literally and also psychologically.

How to delay the onset of dialysis-- at a glance

–   Eat right as well as lose excess weight

- Exercise regularly

- Don't smoke

- Avoid excess salt in your diet

- Control of hypertension

- Control diabetes mellitus

- Stay on the job as well as keep your medical insurance

- Talk with your healthcare team

NUTRITION GUIDE FOR KIDNEY PATIENTS

If you have persistent kidney disease (CKD), it's important to see what you consume. Due to the fact that your kidneys can't get rid of waste items from your body like they should, that's. A kidney-friendly diet regimen can assist you to stay much healthier, much longer.

What's a Kidney-Friendly Diet?

It's a means of consuming that aids shield your kidneys from more damages. It suggests restricting some foods as well as liquids, so certain minerals do not develop in your body. At the very same time, you'll need to make certain you obtain the ideal equilibrium of protein, minerals, calories, and also vitamins.

If you're at the beginning of CKD, there may be few, if any type of, limits on what you can consume. But as your disease becomes worse, you'll need to be more careful regarding what you place into your body.

Your medical professional may suggest you collaborate with a dietitian to pick foods that are easy on your kidneys.

Eating correctly is essential for kidney health and wellness. Individuals with kidney disease need to keep an eye on the consumption of phosphorus, potassium, and sodium, especially.

Individuals with kidney disease might need to control a number of essential nutrients. The complying with info will aid you in adjusting your diet plan.

Please review your particular and individual diet plan requires with your doctor or dietitian.

Right here are some points he may recommend:

Salt

Sodium is a mineral discovered in salt (salt chloride), and also it is widely utilized in cooking. Salt is just one of the most commonly utilized spices, and it requires time to get made use of to lowering the salt in your diet. Nevertheless, reducing salt/sodium is a crucial device in regulating your kidney disease.

- Do not use salt when cooking food.

- Do not place salt on food when you consume.

- Learn to read food tags. Stay clear of foods that have greater than 300mg salt per serving (or 600mg for a full frozen supper). Stay clear of foods that have salt in the very first 4 or 5 products in the component listing.

- Do not consume pork, bacon, sausage, hot canines, luncheon meat, hen tenders or nuggets, or routine tinned soup. Just consume soups that have labels stating the sodium level is lowered-- and also just consume 1 mug-- not the whole can.

- Canned veggies must state "no salt included."

- Do not make use of flavored salts such as garlic salt, onion salt, or "experienced" salt. Likewise, stay clear of kosher or sea salt.

- Be certain to seek lower salt or "no salt added" choices for your favorite foods such as peanut butter or box blends.

- Do not buy icy or refrigerated meats that are packaged "in a solution"; or pre-seasoned/flavored. These items are generally hen breasts, pork chops, pork tenderloin, steaks, or hamburgers.

Potassium

When kidneys do not function properly, potassium develops up in the blood. You will need to stay clear of particular ones and restrict the number of others.

Potassium-rich foods to stay clear of:

- Melons such as melon and also honeydew (watermelon is fine).

- Bananas.

- Oranges as well as orange juice.

- Grapefruit juice.

- Prune juice.

- Tomatoes, tomato sauce, tomato juice.

- Dried beans-- all kinds.

- Pumpkin.

- Winter squash.

- Cooked eco-friendlies, spinach, kale, collards, Swiss Chard.

Other foods to avoid consist of bran grains, granola, "salt replacement" or "lite" salt, molasses. Potatoes, as well as pleasant potatoes, need unique dealing with to allow you to eat them in SMALL quantities.

Be certain to consume a vast range of vegetables and fruits daily to prevent obtaining as well much potassium.

Phosphorus.

When your kidneys don't function properly, phosphorus is another mineral that can develop up in your blood. Calcium can be pulled from your bones and can accumulate in your skin or blood vessels when this happens. The bone conditions can then end up being an issue, making you most likely to have a bone break.

- Dairy foods are the major source of phosphorus in the diet plan, so limit milk to 1 mg per day. , if you use yogurt or cheese instead of fluid milk-- just one container OR 1 ounce a day!

- Some veggies additionally consist of phosphorus. Limit these to 1 mug each week: dried out beans, eco-friendlies, broccoli, mushrooms, and also Brussels sprouts.

- Certain cereals require to be limited to 1 servings a week: bran, wheat cereals, oatmeal, and granola.

- White bread is better than entire grain bread or crackers.

- Soft drinks consist of phosphorus, so just consume clear ones. Do not drink Mountain Dew ® (any kind), sodas, root beers, Dr. Pepper ® (any kind of kind). Prevent Hawaiian Punch ®, Fruitworks ®, Cool ® cold tea, and also Aquafina ® tangerine pineapple.

- Beer likewise has phosphorus-- prevent all kinds.

DIET IN CHRONIC KIDNEY DISEASE

When you have chronic kidney disease (CKD), you may require to make modifications to your diet. These modifications might consist of limiting fluids, eating a low-protein diet, restricting salt, potassium, phosphorus, and other electrolytes, and getting enough calories if you are dropping weight.

You may need to change your diet more if your kidney disease gets worse, or if you require dialysis.

Function

When you have CKD or are on dialysis, the function of this diet plan is to keep the levels of electrolytes, minerals, and fluid in your body stabilized.

Individuals on dialysis need this unique diet plan to restrict the buildup of waste products in the body. Limiting fluids in between dialysis treatments is really crucial due to the fact that the majority of people on dialysis urinate really little. Without urination, fluid will construct up in the body and cause excessive fluid in the heart and lungs.

Recommendations

Ask your healthcare service provider to refer you to a registered dietitian to assist you with your diet for kidney disease. Some dietitians focus on kidney diets. Your dietitian can also help you develop a diet to fit your other health needs.

It is a great place for people with kidney disease and their families to discover programs and info. You require to take in adequate calories each day to keep you healthy and prevent the breakdown of body tissue.

Carbohydrates

If you do not have a problem eating carbs, these foods are an excellent source of energy. If your supplier has actually suggested a low-protein diet plan, you may replace the calories from protein with:

- Fruits, bread, vegetables, and grains. These foods provide energy, in addition to fiber, minerals, and vitamins.

- Hard sweets, jelly, sugar, and honey. If needed, you can even consume high-calorie desserts such as pies, cakes, or cookies, as long as you restrict desserts made with dairy, chocolate, nuts, or bananas.

Fats

Fats can be an excellent source of calories. Make sure to utilize polyunsaturated and monounsaturated fats (olive oil, canola oil, safflower oil) to protect your heart health. Talk with your supplier or dietitian about fats and cholesterol that might increase your risk for heart problems.

Protein

Low-protein diet plans may be handy before you start dialysis. Your provider or dietitian might recommend a lower-protein diet based on your weight, stage of disease, how much muscle you have, and other elements. But you still need enough protein, so work with your provider to find the ideal diet for you.

As soon as you begin dialysis, you will need to consume more protein. A high-protein diet plan with fish, poultry, pork, or eggs at every meal may be suggested.

Individuals on dialysis must eat 8 to 10 ounces (225 to 280 grams) of high-protein foods each day. Your company or dietitian may recommend including egg whites, egg white powder, or protein powder.

Calcium and phosphorous

The minerals calcium and phosphorous will be inspected typically. Even in the early phases of CKD, phosphorus levels in the blood can get too expensive. This can trigger:

- Low calcium. This triggers the body to pull calcium from your bones, which can make your bones weaker and more likely to break.

- Itching.

You will need to restrict the number of dairy foods you consume since they include big amounts of phosphorous. This consists of milk, yogurt, and cheese. Some dairy foods are lower in phosphorous, consisting of:

- Tub margarine

- Butter.

- Cream, ricotta, brie cheese.

- Heavy cream.

- Sherbet.

- Nondairy whipped toppings.

You might require taking calcium supplements to avoid bone disease, and vitamin D to manage the balance of calcium and phosphorus in your body. Ask your supplier or dietitian about how best to get these nutrients.

Your service provider may advise medicines called "phosphorous binders" if diet plan modifications alone do not work to manage the balance of this mineral in your body.

Fluids.

In the early stages of kidney failure, you do not need to restrict the fluid you drink. But, as your condition worsens, or when you are on dialysis, you will require to enjoy the amount of liquid you take in.

In between dialysis sessions, fluid can develop up in the body. Too much fluid will lead to shortness of breath, an emergency situation that needs instant medical attention.

Use smaller sized cups or glasses and turn over your cup after you have actually completed it.

Tips to avoid becoming thirsty include:

- Avoid salty foods.

- Freeze some juice in an ice tray and consume it like a fruit-flavored ice pop (you must count these ice cubes in your day-to-day amount of fluids).

- Stay cool on hot days.

Salt or sodium

Reducing sodium in your diet helps you manage hypertension. It also keeps you from being thirsty and prevents your body from holding onto additional fluid. Try to find these words on food labels:

- Low-sodium.

- No salt added.

- Sodium-free.

- Sodium-reduced.

- Unsalted.

Check all labels to see just how much salt or salty foods include per serving. Likewise, avoid foods that list salt near the start of the active ingredients. Look for items with less than 100 milligrams (mg) of salt per serving.

DO NOT use salt when cooking and take the salt shaker away from the table. Many other herbs are safe, and you can utilize them to taste your food instead of salt.

DO NOT use salt replacements since they include potassium. Individuals with CKD also require to restrict their potassium.

Potassium.

Too much potassium can develop up when the kidneys no longer work well. Fruits and vegetables include large quantities of potassium, and for that reason needs to be avoided to preserve a healthy heart.

Selecting the best item from each food group can assist control your potassium levels.

When consuming fruits:

- Choose peaches, grapes, pears, apples, berries, pineapple, plums, tangerines, and watermelon.

- Limit or avoid oranges and orange juice, nectarines, kiwis, raisins or other dried fruit, bananas, cantaloupe, honeydew, prunes, and nectarines.

When eating vegetables:

- Choose broccoli, cabbage, carrots, cauliflower, celery, cucumber, eggplant, green and wax beans, lettuce, onion, peppers, watercress, zucchini, and yellow squash.

- Limit or avoid asparagus, avocado, potatoes, tomatoes or tomato sauce, winter season squash, pumpkin, avocado, and prepared spinach.

Iron.

People with advanced kidney failure likewise have anemia and normally need additional iron.

Lots of foods consist of extra iron (liver, beef, pork, chicken, lima and kidney beans, iron-fortified cereals). Because of your kidney disease, talk to your service provider or dietitian about which foods with iron you can eat.

RENAL DIET RECIPES

The kidney diet plan (kidney diet) can be among the toughest aspects of living with chronic kidney disease. Not only do you require to determine, with the aid of a dietitian, what foods are excellent (and bad) for you, but then create meals that are pleasing and enjoyable as well. We've compiled a collection of dishes that we discover are yummy however also kidney-friendly. Everyone is different, and each meal might require adjusting depending upon your scenario, so please make sure to talk to your dietitian or medical team if you're unsure about a recipe.

Alaska Baked Macaroni And Cheese

Supper, Entrees, Lunch, Vegetarian, Low Potassium, High Protein, Low Salt

Nutrition Facts per serving

Calories424

Carbohydrates36 g.

Protein22 g.

Dietary Fiber2g.

Fat20g.

Sodium479 mg.

Potassium237 mg.

Phosphorus428 mg.

Sodium: All of our recipes are low in sodium due to the fact that it is tough on kidneys and raises blood pressure. Many people must limit sodium to 1,500 milligrams per day.

Potassium: If you are on hemodialysis, limit potassium too, to 2,000 milligrams per day. Limitation potassium to 3,500 milligrams per day if you are on peritoneal dialysis or brief daily dialysis.

Phosphorus: If you are on dialysis, limit phosphorus to about 1,000 milligrams daily.

Protein: If you are not on dialysis but have kidney disease, you may benefit from a diet lower in protein.

Inspect with a kidney physician or dietitian for standards.

Ingredients

Based on 8 portions per dish.

-   3 cups elbow, little shell, or bowtie pasta.
-   2 tablespoons flour.
-   2 tablespoons unsalted butter.
-   2 cups milk.
-   1 teaspoon mustard powder.
-   1 teaspoon paprika.
-   1 tablespoon fresh thyme or tarragon, chopped or 1 teaspoon dry.
-   2 cups cheese (gouda, cheddar, or any combination).
-   croutons or sliced almonds to taste.

Preparation.

- Heat oven to 350 degrees.

- Boil pasta in a big pot until al-dente.

- Meanwhile, in a medium glass determining cup, measure flour and butter. Microwave about 1-2 minutes until golden brown.

- Slowly stir in milk and continue microwaving up until thickened. Stir in spices and herbs.

- Mix drained pipes noodles, sauce, and cheese and put in a greased casserole dish. Bake about 20 minutes.

- Top with croutons or sliced almonds in the last 5 minutes.

About This Recipe.

A brand-new twist on this traditional dish.

Quick Pesto

Dinner, Sauces, Side Meals, Low Phosphorus, Low Potassium, Low Protein, Low Salt

Nutrition Facts per serving

Calories334

Carbohydrates1 g.

Protein4 g.

Sodium113 mg.

Potassium47 mg.

Phosphorus87 mg.

Sodium: All of our recipes are low in salt since it is tough on kidneys and raises high blood pressure. The majority of people must restrict salt to 1,500 milligrams daily.

Potassium: If you are on hemodialysis, limitation potassium too, to 2,000 milligrams daily. If you are on peritoneal dialysis or short day-to-day dialysis, limit potassium to 3,500 milligrams each day.

Phosphorus: If you are on dialysis, limit phosphorus to about 1,000 milligrams each day.

Protein: If you are not on dialysis however, have kidney disease, you might benefit from a diet lower in protein. Consult a kidney physician or dietitian for standards.

Active ingredients.

Based on 6-8 portions per dish.

- 40 fresh basil leaves.
- 1 garlic clove.
- 2 tablespoons walnuts.
- 10 tablespoons grated parmesan cheese.
- 2/3 cup olive oil.

Preparation.

- Process all ingredients except the oil in food processor or mixer until fine.

- With motor running, slowly include oil until well mixed.

- Enjoy hot pasta.

About This Recipe.

Fresh pesto is tasty on pasta, pizza, or a sandwich.

BBQ Rub For Pork Or Chicken

Flavorings, Low Phosphorus, Low Potassium, Low Protein, Low Salt

Nutrition Facts per serving

Calories20

Carbohydrates4 g.

Protein0 g.

Dietary Fiber0 g.

Sodium9 mg.

Potassium34 mg.

Phosphorus7 mg.

Salt: All of our recipes are low in sodium since it is hard on kidneys and raises high blood pressure. The majority of people need to restrict sodium to 1,500 milligrams daily.

Potassium: If you are on hemodialysis, limitation potassium too, to 2,000 milligrams daily. If you are on peritoneal dialysis or brief daily dialysis, limit potassium to 3,500 milligrams each day.

Phosphorus: If you are on dialysis, limit phosphorus to about 1,000 milligrams per day.

Protein: If you are not on dialysis but have kidney disease, you might benefit from a diet plan lower in protein. Contact a kidney medical professional or dietitian for guidelines.

Ingredients .

Based on 4 servings per dish.

- 1 tablespoon brown sugar.
- 1 teaspoon smoked paprika.
- 1 teaspoon chili powder.
- 1 teaspoon garlic, granulated.
- 1 teaspoon onion powder.
- 1 teaspoon cumin.
- 1/4 teaspoon dry mustard powder.
- 1/8 teaspoon allspice.
- 1/8 teaspoon ground red pepper (optional).

Preparation.

- In a bowl, blend all active ingredients together completely.

- Rub on pork or chicken prior to cooking.

About This Recipe.

Get innovative and make your own salt totally free BBQ mix.

40-Second Omelet

Breakfast, Low Phosphorus, Low Potassium, High Protein, Low Sodium

Nutrition Facts per serving

Calories255

Carbohydrates1.3 g.

Protein13 g.

Dietary Fiber2 g.

Sodium145 mg.

Potassium122 mg.

Phosphorus195 mg.

Sodium: All of our dishes are low in sodium since it is difficult on kidneys and raises high blood pressure. Many people must limit sodium to 1,500 milligrams per day.

Potassium: If you are on hemodialysis, limitation potassium too, to 2,000 milligrams each day. Limitation potassium to 3,500 milligrams per day if you are on peritoneal dialysis or short everyday dialysis.

Phosphorus: If you are on dialysis, limitation phosphorus to about 1,000 milligrams daily.

Protein: If you are not on dialysis; however, have kidney disease, you might take advantage of a diet plan lower in protein. Talk to a kidney physician or dietitian for standards.

Ingredients

Based on 1 serving per dish.

- 2 eggs.
- 2 tablespoons water.
- 1 tablespoon unsalted butter.
- 1/2 cup filling (veggie, meat, seafood).

Preparation.

- Beat together eggs and water till combined.

- In a 10-inch omelet pan or frying pan, heat butter up until just hot adequate to sizzle a drop of water.

- Pour in the egg mix. The mixture should set at edges right now. With an inverted pancake turner, thoroughly push prepared portions at edges toward center so uncooked parts can reach the hot pan surface area. Tilt pan and move as needed.

- Continue up until egg is set and will not stream. Fill the omelet with 1/2 cup of vegetable, seafood, fruit, or meat filling, if preferred. If you're ideal handed and the ideal side, if you're left-handed, put filling on left side.

- With the pancake turner, fold omelet in half. Invert onto a plate with the omelet's bottom side dealing with up.

About This Recipe.

Eggs are an excellent source of protein and a fast meal when time is restricted.

60-Second Salsa

Sauces, Vegetarian, Low Phosphorus, Low Potassium, Low Protein, Low Sodium

Nutrition Facts per serving

Calories14

Carbohydrates2 g.

Protein1 g.

Dietary Fiber0 g.

Fat1 g.

Sodium4 mg.

Potassium117 mg.

Phosphorus14 mg.

Salt: All of our dishes are low in sodium because it is tough on kidneys and raises high blood pressure. A lot of individuals need to limit salt to 1,500 milligrams per day.

Potassium: If you are on hemodialysis, limitation potassium too, to 2,000 milligrams daily. If you are on peritoneal dialysis or short everyday dialysis, limitation potassium to 3,500 milligrams per day.

Phosphorus: If you are on dialysis, limitation phosphorus to about 1,000 milligrams daily.

Protein: If you are not on dialysis; however, have kidney disease, you might benefit from a diet lower in protein. Check with a kidney doctor or dietitian for guidelines.

Ingredients.

Based on 8 portions per recipe.

- 4 roma or plum tomatoes, sliced.
- 2 green onions, chopped.
- 3 garlic cloves, minced.
- 1/2 - 1 green bell pepper, sliced.
- 1/2 - 1 fresh jalapeño, sliced.
- 1/2 lot fresh cilantro, chopped.
- 1/2 teaspoon cumin.
- 1/4 cup fresh oregano, sliced or 1 tablespoon dried.

Preparation.

- Mix all components in a food processor or blender up until the bigger products are chunky and small.

- Let sit for a couple of hours in the refrigerator.

- Best served chilled and with plain tortilla chips.

About This Recipe.

Use fresh summertime veggies to work up this scrumptious salsa.

Do not go yet; One last thing yo do...

If you enjoyed this book or found it useful, I'd be very grateful if you'd post a short review on **Amazon**. Your support does make a difference, and I read all the reviews personally so I can get your feedback and make this book even better.

Thanks again for your support!

© Copyright 2019 by **SIMON LEE**